THE ESSENCE OF YOGA

THE ESSENCE OF YOGA

Essays on the Development of Yogic Philosophy from the Vedas to Modern Times

GEORG FEUERSTEIN
AND JEANINE MILLER

Inner Traditions International
Rochester, Vermont

Inner Traditions International
One Park Street
Rochester, Vermont 05767
www.gotoit.com

First Inner Traditions edition published 1998

Originally published in Great Britain under the title *A Reappraisal of Yoga*

Library of Congress Cataloging-in-Publication Data

Feuerstein, Georg.
[Reappraisal of yoga]
The essence of yoga : essays on the development of yogic philosophy from the Vedas to modern times / Georg Feuerstein and Jeanine Miller.
p. cm.
Originally published: London : Rider, 1971, under title: A reappraisal of yoga; published: New York : Schocken, 1972, under title: Yoga and beyond.
Includes bibliographical references and index.
ISBN 0-89281-738-0 (pbk. : alk. paper)
1. Yoga. I. Miller, Jeanine. II. Title.
B132.Y6F48 1997 97-13386
181'.45—dc21 CIP

Printed and bound in the United States

10 9 8 7 6 5 4 3 2 1

Distributed to the book trade in Canada by Publishers Group West (PGW), Toronto, Ontario
Distributed to the book trade in the United Kingdom by Deep Books, London
Distributed to the book trade in Australia by Millennium Books, Newtown, N.S.W.
Distributed to the book trade in New Zealand by Tandem Press, Auckland
Distributed to the book trade in South Africa by Alternative Books, Ferndale

Acknowledgements

Our thanks are due to the authors and publishers for permission to quote from the following works:

A. J. Toynbee, *A Study of History*, vol. III, Oxford University Press, London.

R. Otto, *Mysticism: East & West*, Collier-Macmillan Ltd., London.

A. Montagu, *The Concept of the Primitive*, The Free Press, New York.

T. Dobzhansky, *The Biology of Ultimate Concern*, Rapp & Whiting, London.

D. T. Suzuki, *Mysticism: Christian and Buddhist*, Allen & Unwin, London.

A. Eddington, *Science and the Unseen*, Allen & Unwin.

A. Huxley, *The Perennial Philosophy*, W. Collins Sons & Co., London.

Shree Purohit Swami, *Aphorisms of Yoga*, Faber & Faber, London.

E. Underhill, *Mysticism. A Study in the Nature & Development of Man's Spiritual Consciousness*, Methuen & Co., London.

M. Eliade, *Yoga: Immortality & Freedom*, Routledge & Kegan Paul, London.

M. Eliade, *Shamanism*, Bollingen Foundation, New York.

R. C. Zaehner, *Mysticism: Sacred & Profane*, Clarendon Press, London.

J. Ellistone, *The Signature of All Things*, Dent & Son, London.

L. Renou, *Religions of Ancient India*, Schocken Books, New York.

Elmer O'Brien, *The Essential Plotinus*, New American Library, New York.

J. Gonda, *The Vision of the Vedic Poets*, Mouton & Co., The Hague, Netherlands.

S. S. Suryanarayana Sastri, *The Bhamati*, Theosophical Publishing House, Adyar, India.

Shri Aurobindo, *On the Veda*, Shri Aurobindo Ashram, Pondicherry, India.

A. B. Purani, *Sri Aurobindo's Vedic Glossary*, Shri Aurobindo Ashram.

V. S. Agrawala, *Sparks from the Vedic Fire*, School of Vedic Studies, Varanasi, India.

J. Gebser, *Ursprung & Gegenwart*, Deutsche Verlagsanstalt, Stuttgart, Germany.

J. Quint, *Meister Eckehart*, Carl Hanser Verlag, München, Germany.

Portions of the essay on Agni and the note on Ṛgvedic interpretation were published in *Hinduism*, Journal of the Bharat Sevashram Sangha, London Branch.

Contents

Abbreviations

BhG	=	Bhagavad-Gītā
Bṛh. Up.	=	Bṛhadāraṇyaka-Upaniṣad
Ṛgv.	=	Ṛgveda(-Saṃhitā)
TV	=	Tattva-Vaiśāradī
Up.	=	Upaniṣad
YBh.	=	Yoga-Bhāṣya
YS	=	Yoga-Sūtra

These abbreviations are restricted to the footnotes and used in the main text only when in a secondary position. Other abbreviations are obvious.

Preface

It is our deep conviction that the discoveries and insights of Yoga are of the highest significance for a proper understanding of the human situation in general and the present state of affairs in particular. The change taking place in Western culture, the effects of which can clearly be perceived in all cultural domains, harbours seedlings of a new spirituality that need to be awakened and attended to if we wish to overcome the steadily spreading crisis of man which, as Jean Gebser observes, is 'not a mere crisis of morals, economics, ideologies, politics, religion', but a global crisis.[1] In this connection we wish to quote Simone Weil, the French mystic and scientist, who wrote: 'If the crisis of our age is comparable to that of the fifth century B.C. then there is an obvious duty; to make another effort comparable to that of Eudoxus.'[2] The problems which we have to face today are, whether we like it or not, of a profound *religious* nature or, to put it differently, are related to man as the heir to transcendent reality. The same questions that concern us at present perturbed man in India many centuries ago in a very similar way. It is axiomatic therefore that we should give serious attention to Indian spirituality, however strange the formulations and solutions of the Eastern mind may seem to us at first. We cannot afford to ignore the psychological-cum-philosophical findings of the old Indian culture which reached a high religious and philosophical maturity at an early time and which, on account of its rich experiences over more than four millennia, can be of incomparable help in the present struggle of Western man.

Our special attention must be paid to Yoga, for it is in a way the most precious concentrate of all the spiritual riches of India. Its true value has hardly been recognised in the Western world. This is mainly

[1] J. Gebser, *Ursprung und Gegenwart* (Stuttgart, 1966), p. xix.
[2] S. Weil, *Seventy Letters* (London, Oxford University Press, 1965), p. 91.

due to the fact that from the beginning Yoga was seen, both by scholars and others concerned with it, from an outside point of view. Apart from a few exceptions, there has been little genuine endeavour to follow the Yogic path and to test its methods and verify its statements experimentally. The German physician and depth psychologist Dr. H. Speer bluntly stated that the scientists wishing to approach the real nature of Yoga must submit themselves to its practical application at least for a few years.[3] This reminds us of a maxim in Vyāsa's commentary to the *Yoga-Sūtra* which states: 'Yoga has to be known by Yoga. Yoga manifests through Yoga.'[4] Let us also not forget William James' words quoted by A. Huxley: 'Practice may change our theoretical horizon, and this in a twofold way: it may lead into new worlds and secure new powers.'[5] Western man loves to theorise and likes to withdraw from practice. Although almost two hundred years ago Kant had by way of logic shown that the intellect is not capable of solving the deeper metaphysical problems, what could be called the jungle of Western metaphysics is nevertheless steadily continuing to expand.

In Yoga metaphysical questions play a minor role. To the yogin philosophy is never the final object; his aim is to actually 'experience' that which for Kant was the everlasting object of human mind, the reality beyond the phenomenal world. Long before the *Critique of Pure Reason* was written, yogins in the East had recognised the insufficiency of the intellect with regard to the cognition of final truths. They did not, however, fall into the fatal error of overlooking this fact in their statement of the problem of man's nature, as is generally the case nowadays, but they sought after a 'faculty' in man which might break through the limits of the mind. And, as they assure us again and again in their writings, they have discovered a way—the method of Yoga. Even if we are not willing or prepared to follow Yoga up to its very heights, a profound theoretical *and* practical study of it would undoubtedly lead to many a remarkable discovery, particularly in the fields of psychology, depth psychology and parapsychology which may well be called sciences of the future.

Yoga, if unlocked by personal practice, could prove to be of a far greater value towards a re-moulding of human personality and thus of our age than any other science, religion or philosophy, for it opens to us

[3] *Vide* H. Speer's preface to E. Haich, *Sexuelle Kraft und Yoga* (Stuttgart, 1966).
[4] YBh III. 6.
[5] A. Huxley, *The Perennial Philosophy*, 3rd impr. (London, Glasgow, 1961), p. 10.

a completely new aspect of existence—the realm of the Self beyond personality and phenemonal world.

The present book is, as the title suggests, a collection of essays endeavouring to portray the living pulse of Indian philosophy, the art and science of Yoga. Stress was laid on a general appraisal or, rather, reappraisal of this extremely ancient teaching. The introductory essay is meant to give an outline of Yoga, particularly in its classical form. We have dwelt at length upon the central technique of Yoga, the practice of *samādhi* or enstasis, often misleadingly called ecstasy. In this connection we have especially treated the question of the succession of the diverse enstatic grades according to classical Yoga—a theme which has hitherto been greatly misrepresented. The second essay is a prelude to the subsequent articles on ancient Indian spirituality. It gives out the basic principles of our attempts at interpreting the Vedas, particularly the *Ṛgveda*, which is the fountain-head of all later Indian systems of thought. As already stated by H. D. Griswold, no real understanding of later Hinduism is possible without a knowledge of the probably oldest literary monument of mankind, the *Ṛgveda*.[6] This is particularly true of Yoga, the basic practices and conceptions of which can be traced back to this archaic scripture. To show this is the aim of the essays on (i) the *keśin-sūkta* which contains references to very old notions and practices showing great similarity to those of later Yoga, on (ii) the hymn of creation (*nāsadīya-sūkta*) which foreshadows the ontological teachings of the epic and classical Yoga-Sāṃkhya traditions, and on (iii) Agni, the grand figure of the *Ṛgveda*, who heralds the Upaniṣadic *ātman* as well as the Tantric 'serpent fire' or *kuṇḍalinī*. The fourth essay, on the meaning of suffering in Yoga, considers the basic issue of the philosophy underlying classical Yoga: suffering and its termination. The concluding essay is on Meister Eckehart's spiritual teachings, which show a striking resemblance to the most advanced philosophical schools of India.

We have quoted extensively from the Sanskrit originals and are, when not stated otherwise, responsible for all the renderings. In our essay on Agni, however, we have made use of Griffith's poetical translation of the Ṛgvedic hymns without explicitly stating so. All renderings from German and French are ours.

G.F. and J.M.

London, 1970

[6] *Vide* H. D. Griswold, *The Religion of the Rigveda* (London, 1923), p. 328.

THE ESSENCE OF
YOGA

I The Essence of Yoga

As indicated in the preface, the nucleus of Yoga is its practice, and the yogin is primarily practitioner, not philosopher, theologist or psychologist in the common sense. In his radical practical approach he is comparable to the scientist who spends most of his time not at his desk, but in the laboratory. The yogin is not satisfied with theorising, guessing or accepting facts second hand—he takes his own experience (*pratyakṣa* or 'perception') as the highest criterion. This is all the more necessary as his object of study is not only the most sublime, but also the most difficult a man can choose. The yogin's aim is the realisation of the transcendent reality or, in the words of Kant, the thing-in-itself[1] behind and beyond the world of appearances, which for the yogin is naturally neither fictitious nor alien to experience. Kant, however, would not admit the possibility of the latter, because he discarded what generally and less precisely is referred to as 'mystical experience'. But R. Otto, commenting on Kant's distinction between the empirical knowledge as gained through sense-impressions and as attained by pure reason, says: 'The numinous is of the latter kind. . . . The proof that in the numinous we have to deal with purely *a priori* cognitive elements is to be reached by introspection and a critical examination of reason such as Kant instituted.'[2] For the yogin actual realisation of the ultimate reality is not mere sensing, but direct experience or *sākṣātkāra*; he regards it as a possibility open to everyone. All that is required is a radical devotion to the practical application (*abhyāsa*) of Yoga. This is but natural. Even the scientist having made certain discoveries will, when demonstrating his experiments, do it under the original laboratory conditions. If the experiment is repeated by someone not keeping

[1] *sva-lakṣaṇa* in Sanskrit.

[2] R. Otto, *The Idea of the Holy*, transl. by J. W. Harvey (Harmondsworth, 1959), p. 130.

to these conditions, it will certainly not be the fault of the scientist if completely irrelevant results are obtained. This is particularly true of Yoga. To come to a really objective conclusion about its aim, purpose and value, one must subject oneself to the 'experimental conditions' demanded by the yogins, that is, one has to follow their techniques, practices and instructions point by point.

He who really wishes to penetrate deeper into Yoga and come to a just appreciation of it cannot avoid studying the inner and outer basis from which it evolved. Many phenomena are only intelligible when viewed in the light of the most recent research in history, comparative sciences, anthropology and last but not least psychology. Only in this way can numerous methods and doctrines of Yoga be saved from the reproach of being worthless products of primitive magical-cum-mythical thought. It is therefore necessary to give a brief outline of the cultural background of Yoga and to explain its teaching and practice in connection with the whole religious culture of man.

The germ of Yoga doubtlessly is the inborn human longing to cross the threshold of this phenomenal world, which Meister Eckehart expressed in the following words: 'Know that all creatures pursue and act, by nature, to the end to become like God.'[3] The Buddha, almost two thousand years earlier, compared this urge, expressing itself more or less impetuously, with an arrow in one's heart which can only be removed by knowledge—transcendental knowledge, *prajñā* or *γνῶσις*. The conviction that there is something that surpasses reality as we know it and that is immanent in man, Ibn Khaldūn, the famous fourteenth-century Arabic historian, described thus:

> The human soul has an innate disposition to divest itself of its human nature in order to clothe itself in the nature of the angels and to become an angel in reality for a single instant of time—a moment which comes and goes as swiftly as the flicker of an eyelid. Thereupon the soul resumes its human nature, after having received, in the world of angels, a message which it has to carry to its own human kind.[4]

[3] Sermon 40. Edited and translated into German by J. Quint, *Meister Eckehart. Deutsche Predigten und Traktate* (München, 1955).

[4] A. J. Toynbee, *A Study of History*, vol. III (London, Oxford University Press, 1934), p. 249. The rendering is based on the French translation of Khaldūn's *Muquaddamat* by Baron M. G. de Slane (*Histoire des Berbères* p. 437).

This strange 'disposition' towards metaphysical experience can only be understood from man's past which, in fact, gives us the key to a comprehension of the present human situation. (The great interest of our time in the extinct cultures of the East, Europe, and South America seems to derive its impulse from the urgent desire that from there insights may be gained which are able to cast light upon the entangled situation of modern life. Curiosity alone cannot explain this distinct tendency.)

How deep the bearing of human past really is, the cultural studies of the Swiss scholar Jean Gebser have revealed. They have disclosed that humanity, in the course of its evolution, traversed diverse stages of consciousness which are still present in us in a latent state and, indeed, *constitute* us. J. Gebser detected four such structures or, as he terms them, 'mutations' of consciousness in the past and found indications of a fifth structure which he styles 'integral consciousness'. The 'level' most close to the beginning (not origin, for it is transcendent), or even identical with it, is the 'archaic' consciousness, 'the time where the soul is still asleep'.[5] It is followed by the 'magical', the 'mythical' and the 'mental' mutations. All four structures are well documented and analysed in a most understanding and farseeing way. For our present purpose, it will suffice to quote two sentences from Gebser's voluminous work: 'Magical man possessed not only the ability of television and tele-audition, but he was also highly telepathical.'[6]

And: 'The Aura drawings [for example those in Australia] make it clear that the faculty of perception in early man was different from ours: he saw partly more and partly less than we do today. Anyway, he saw emanations of force, saw the moving power; he saw part of the Mana of a person.'[7]

These abilities, forming part of the psychomental constitution of man at the dawn of history, disappeared due to the growing awakening to the physical world and himself. Even today, relics of this ancient structure of consciousness—indicating that it is still in us—can be found in a few especially sensitive persons, so-called mediums, in whom these faculties of mind come into action spontaneously. More rarely these abilities manifest themselves by hallucinogenic drugs.[8] These

[5] J. Gebser, *Ursprung und Gegenwart* p. 52.
[6] op. cit., p. 66.
[7] op. cit., p. 222.
[8] We would like to draw attention to a very conclusive account of such an

phenomena not only strengthen Gebser's view on the strange psychomental constitution of early man, but also leave no doubt about the fact that these old types of consciousness are still in us and active, either overtly or covertly. In Yoga they are a very common and, one may say, regular feature of the practical realisation or *sādhana*. However, in true Yoga no special meaning is attributed to them, and they are regarded as being mere 'waste-products' of the meditative efforts. 'These [abilities] are perfections to the emergent [or waking consciousness] [but] obstacles in the enstasis.'[9] This critical attitude towards magical powers (*siddhis*, *vibhūtis*) is a fact not to be overlooked, for it points out that Yoga proper is not a falling back into any of the primitive forms of consciousness.

These findings clearly are of utmost significance for religion in general and for Yoga, drawing from the same sources, in particular, because the psychomental constitution of early man *empirically* explains why the religious sphere—as depth psychology has shown and as especially C. G. Jung has set clear—plays such an all-important role even in the life of modern man. In the archaic stage of human evolution, man was in direct contact with the 'heavens'.[10] However, this contact was not a conscious one, for man had not yet developed either world- or self-consciousness. J. Gebser therefore equates this state with deep sleep in which, according to Vedānta, an unconscious merging into the Absolute takes place. It is these conditions in prehistory which form the foundation of all religion. Since the individual is composed of all the structures of consciousness through which the human race strode during its evolution, he also possesses a 'memory' of the basic tone of the archaic state which expresses itself in the more or less conscious longing to regain this 'forfeit' dimension of existence, the state before the 'fall'. Thus the basis of religion is neither wishful thinking nor mere speculation about the inexplicable, nor is it modified sexual energy. Rather it is the manifestation of the urge to win anew the 'lost paradise', the former 'kingdom of heaven', to make use of the Christian phraseology. However, we hasten to add that this re-linking sought by religion is not simply a reinstatement of the original archaic condition.

instance by a University professor quoted in R. C. Johnson, *Watcher on the Hills* (London, 1959?), pp. 157–60.

[9] YS III.37: *te samādhāv-upasargā vyutthāne siddhayaḥ.*

[10] This is also the main instruction to be derived from the so-called 'paradisiac' myths occurring all over the world.

It cannot be, for the 're-turn' must, by nature, be a conscious one, otherwise the destination will be . . . deep sleep. Religion and also Yoga must be understood as a 'returning home' to the origin (*Ursprung*) which is transcendent and not to the temporal beginning (*Anfang*) or initial *empirical* structure of consciousness. This distinction is of serious consequence, for there is all the difference in the world between the archaic state of consciousness, the manifested or human consciousness, which is the object of anthropological or historical studies, and that consciousness which *is* the transcendent reality, *cit* as *sat*. Yoga cannot be characterised as a regressing to primitive types of consciousness, be it that of the archaic, mythical or magical structure. The Yogic process of transformation (*pratipakṣa*) is in all its parts and phases a conscious involution which ends in a supraconscious illumination (*prajñā*) and not, as prejudiced and uninformed critics usually maintain, in a cataleptic state or, as some cynics hold, in a deep sleep. The Yogic 'state' is, in Vedāntic circles, called the 'fourth (*turīya*), simply because it differs from the three empirical states of consciousness, namely waking (*jāgrat*), dream sleep (*svapna*) and deep sleep (*suṣupti*). The last would be properly attributed to the original state of *human* consciousness which J. Gebser classifies as null-dimensional, perspective-less, pre-spacial and pre-temporal.

As explained above, religion and Yoga are both grounded on the concrete experience of the numinous—a term coined by R. Otto—in the earliest history of man, but while the former is more of the nature of a reflex, a spontaneous reaction to the subconscious spiritual needs, the latter is predominantly, if not exclusively, rationalistic in so far as it makes these subconscious spiritual stimuli fully conscious and responds to them with a full-fledged scheme for their realisation or fulfilment. In Yoga this dynamic spiritual urge is recognised as the motive behind all human activities which can only be satisfied by the actual realisation of the ultimate reality. This is what St. Augustine meant when he said: 'Thou hast created us for Thy sake, and our heart is ever restless till it finds rest in Thee.'[11]

The nostalgia for the original consciousness, as opposed to the primary empirical state of mind which is the transcendent *cit* under the veil of the universal *māyā*, must, at an early time, have led to certain practices which were intended to re-link (*religare*) with the 'yonder world'. From here to a systematic training cannot have been a step too

[11] *Confessions* I.1.

big. One thing is certain, the beginnings of Yoga are not to be connected with the practical testing of a learned doctrine, as J. Filliozat maintained, when considering the doctrine of *prāṇa* as the starting point of Yoga.[12] That would mean putting the cart in front of the horse! We entirely agree with J. W. Hauer who recognised that the older or basic elements of Yoga were, in a way, common knowledge of early humanity.[13]

The scientist wishing to give a precise definition of the term *yoga* would fail on account of the complexity of the subject on the one hand and by reason of the incompleteness of our thematical and historical knowledge on the other. He must be satisfied with approximations and descriptive circumscriptions. Probably the shortest 'definition' ever given is found in Vyāsa's *Bhāṣya* on the *Yoga-Sūtra*; he states succinctly: 'Yoga=enstasis.'[14] This formula, even if it cannot be looked upon as a proper definition, is correct and fraught with meaning and far more precise than the usual explanations of the word as 'Indian philosophical system' or similar. For Yoga we cannot employ such terms as 'philosophy', 'psychology' or 'religion' without making certain restrictions. None of these terms can do full justice to the nature of Yoga. Indeed, it contains aspects of all three disciplines, but it exceeds them too. To the Greek 'love of wisdom' (φιλοσοφία) it adds the physical and psychomental practice, widens the 'knowledge about the soul' (ψυχολογία) to a metapsychology,[15] and supplements the religious

[12] J. Filliozat, 'Les origines d'une technique mystique indienne', *Revue philosophique*, 1946 (Paris), p. 217f.

[13] J. W. Hauer, *Der Yoga. Ein indischer Weg zum Selbst*, 2nd enl. ed. (Stuttgart, 1958), p. 19f. J. W. Hauer who passed away in 1966 was a pupil of R. Garbe to whom we owe a great deal in the study of Yoga and Sāṃkhya. J. W. Hauer not only possessed a rich knowledge of Indian thought, but was also well acquainted with Western culture, as the selection of titles below will convey. The central theme of all his works is man as religious being, and Hauer himself was a sincere god-seeker and mystic. Besides his books on Yoga, he also wrote: *Die Religionen. Ihr Werden, ihr Sinn, ihre Wahrheit* (Stuttgart, 1923); *Glaubensgeschichte der Indogermanen*, vol. I (Stuttgart, 1927); *Der abendländische Mensch* (Stuttgart, 1964?), and many more.

[14] *yogaḥ samādhiḥ*. (YBh. I.1.)

[15] This word is here used not in the sense of Freud's psychological interpretation as something which in other sciences is called 'general theory', but in the meaning given to it by J. W. Hauer who introduced the term in order to distinguish between the empirically not accessible 'dynamic preconditions' of the psychomental processes from their underlying physical acts.

sensing and feeling with a radical exercising of the mind with the aim of realising the transcendent reality by immediate perception—an act in which the empirical subject–object relationship is transcended and 'pure consciousness' (*cin-mātra*) or, as Patañjali would express it, the 'power behind the mind' (*citi-śakti*) rests in itself, whereby the word *śakti* stands for the transcendent Self. In the native *Ṛgveda-Saṃhitā* the metaphysical realisation is again and again referred to by the word *dhī* and its derivatives. This family of words was for long left unfathomed by Western indologists, but has now found an able examiner in J. Gonda.[16]

A. W. Watts attempted to explain Yoga as a sort of psychotherapy, but made the common mistake of estimating on a purely psychological level.[17] There is doubtlessly a great similarity between Yoga and psychotherapy. However, the former does not stop at a mere 'integration' or, as some prefer to call it, 'actualisation' of the psyche; it aims at nothing less than a *complete transformation* of man. This will have to be elucidated. The purpose of psychotherapy is, as we understand it, to fully restore the capacity of functioning of a person, to free him from mental duresses and to make him mature emotionally and in his social relationships. Usually the person undergoing psychotherapy is afflicted with certain negative dispositions, physically and mentally. In other words, he comes to the psychotherapist as a patient. Yoga, on the contrary, generally starts with the normal, healthy individual. This fact is made quite plain in the Sanskrit texts: 'The Self is not to be gained by the weak.'[18] And in the *Mahābhārata*, the grand Indian epic, we can read that '. . . the vow of Yoga is only for a man of unweakened mind, for none else that is clear'.[19] Numerous other passages, to the same effect, are to be found particularly in the scriptures of Haṭhayoga and Tantrism. Yoga starting with the mentally and physically 'normal' person can never be an arena for neurotics or psychopaths. It is symptomatic that in the West Haṭhayoga is promoted as a system of health although, in its classical form, it makes physical and psychomental fitness a basic requirement for its practice.

The starting point of Yoga being already different from that of psychotherapy, its aims are still more dissimilar. Yoga commences with

[16] J. Gonda, *The Vision of the Vedic Poets* (The Hague, 1963), pp. 68–169.

[17] A. W. Watts, *Psychotherapy East and West* (New York, 1961).

[18] *Muṇḍaka-Upaniṣad* III.2.

[19] MBh. XII.308.12.

a person sound in every respect and has in view not a restoration to normality or an amelioration of functioning or adaptation, but a man's emancipation from all restrictions peculiar to a human being. That is, it intends to restore man as a transcendent entity. Accordingly, this emancipation is based on a transmutation of human nature. M. Eliade, leading authority in the field of the history of religions and benevolent critic of Yoga, has carried out a profound analysis of this basic phenomenon of spiritual life.[20] He characterised the Yogic path as a progressive dismantling of human personality ending in a complete abolition. With every step (*aṅga*) of Yoga what we call 'man' is demolished a little more. This is in fact what the mystics of all ages and countries taught. To quote but a few examples from the Christian tradition. Meister Eckehart, the great German seer-philosopher of the 13th century (and a contemporary of Rāmānanda, famous expounder of Rāmānuja's Viśiṣṭādvaita-Vedānta), writes in his *Reden der Unterweisung* (§4): 'As much as you go out of all things that much, not more and not less, God enters with all of his, insofar as you in all things completely give up what is yours.'[21] In another piece of writing referring to the 'noble man' (*homo nobilis*) he, after having divided the spiritual path into six steps, describes the last in the following way:

> It is the sixth step when man is dis-formed and super-formed by God's eternity and has reached to wholly perfect forgetting of the transitory and temporal life and is gone and transformed into a godly picture, when he has become the child of God. Still higher and above this there is no step, and there is eternal peace and bliss, for the final aim of the inner man and new man is eternal life.[22]

Angelus Silesius, a speculative mystic of the 17th century, teaches in his *Cherubischer Wandersmann*: 'The more you can empty and pour out yourself of yourself, the more God has to flow into you with his

[20] M. Eliade, *Yoga: Immortality and Freedom*, transl. by W. R. Trask (London, 1958).

[21] This and all following translations of Eckehart's writings are based on the German edition by J. Quint, *Meister Eckehart. Deutsche Predigten und Traktate* (München, 1955). The numbering of the sermons is also his.

[22] *Vom edlen Menschen.* We have deliberately tried to give as much a literal rendering as possible in order to enable the English reader to catch a glimpse of the peculiar philosophical style of the German original.

god-ness.' A. Huxley quotes an interesting passage from Benet of Canfield who, describing the engraved frontispiece of the edition of *The Rule of Perfection*, explains:

> The light of the divine will shines but little on the faces of the first circle of souls living in the divine will; much more on those of the second; while those of the third or innermost circle are resplendent. The features of the first show up most clearly; the second, less; the third, hardly at all. This signifies that the souls of the first degree are much in themselves; those of the second degree are less in themselves and more in God; those in the third degree are almost nothing in themselves and all in God, absorbed in his essential will.[23]

Man, as we have stated at the beginning of this essay, is fundamentally a transcendent entity, a fact which, by Thomas à Kempis, was given the following poetical expression: 'What do you seek here, since this world is not your resting place? Your true home is in Heaven.'[24] Therefore, the path leading to the goal is, as seen from a negative empirical standpoint, a total opposition to life[25] or, as viewed from a positive empirical standpoint, an imitation of reality in its manifested form as the cosmos and then an identification with or merging into its 'own state' (*sva-rūpa*). The former viewpoint is naturally the more weighty one, for it constitutes the actual techniques of the spiritual transformation, while the latter is, concretely speaking, more or less the result of these efforts. M. Eliade discriminates between three major phases of this transformatory process, calling them the 'cosmicisation', the 'recasting of man in new, gigantic dimensions' and the 'final withdrawal' respectively.[26] The first phase is covered by all practices from the ethical precepts (*yama* and *niyama*) up to the meditative concentration (*dhyāna*). With the enstatic state (*samādhi*), man enters into the 'macran-

[23] A. Huxley, *The Perennial Philosophy*, 3rd impr. (London and Glasgow, 1961), p. 59.

[24] *De imitatione Christi* II.1, transl. by Leo Sherley-Price. *The Imitation of Christ*, 3rd ed. (Harmondsworth, 1956).

[25] But to prevent foregone conclusions, we have to state here that *true* Indian spirituality never, at any time, displayed an inclination to *de*valuate life. 'The touch of the Earth is always reinvigorating to the son of Earth, even when he seeks a supra-physical knowledge.' Aurobindo, *The Life Divine* (Pondicherry, 1953), p. 13.

[26] *Vide* M. Eliade, *Yoga: Immortality and Freedom*, p. 98.

thropical' stage. For reasons of clarity we choose to differ here from M. Eliade's terminology, in so far as we speak of a two-phase cosmicisation, a physical and a supraphysical. In the first phase the yogin imitates the empirical universe, in the second he, through the power of *samādhi*, identifies himself with the subtle or *sūkṣma* (Lt. *subtīlis*) aspects constituting the 'fourth dimension' or the 'spiritual depth' of the cosmos. But to reach the transcendent reality, the 'wholly other' (*Ganz Andere*),[27] he has to abandon any form of cosmic existence whatsoever. This includes, as Patañjali and all other philosopher-yogins assure us, the many heavenly regions or *svarga-lokas*. That the heavens, as the abodes of the gods (*devas*), or, in Christian phraseology, the angels, are still within the range of the manifested cosmos and thus subject to birth, death and rebirth has, for example, also been discerned by Eckehart and Jakob Böhme. The former declares: 'The noblest creatures are the angels, and they are purely spiritual and have no corporeality in themselves, and of them exist most, and they are more than the totality of all physical things.'[28] Yet they are *creatures* and as such, in the eyes of the Meister, a 'mere naught' (*bloss niht*). Even God as creative principle or δημιουργός, which in India is given the name *brahma* (masc.) or *īśvara*,[29] is to be exceeded. This distinction can already be encountered in the *Ṛgveda*, as when the seer of the *nāsadīya-sūkta* (X.129) employs the demonstrative pronoun *sa*(*ḥ*) or 'he' when referring to God as the author of the world and *ta*(*t*) or 'it' with regard to the impersonal Absolute. This is in complete line with such Western spiritual heroes as Plotinus, Eckehart and Ruysbroeck; the Meister, for instance, declares: '. . . my essential being is above God insofar as we take God as the beginning of all creatures'.[30] For him God in his triple nature as father, son and Holy Ghost is not the ultimate principle, since beyond him is the 'silent desert', the Godhead, the unutterable, nameless and formless One which is not different from man's Self, the *bürgelin* or apex of the soul. Thus to speak paradoxically and in Eckehart's very own words, God is a non-God. F. H. Bradley came, by way of logic, to the same conclusion: 'We may say that God is not God, till he has become all in all, and that a God which is all in all is not the God of

[27] *Cf.* *Śvetāśvatara-Up.* (V.1): 'He who reigns over knowledge (*vidyā*) is the Other.'

[28] Sermon 4. *Cf.* sermons 3, 39, 56 and 57.

[29] Here not the 'lord' of the YS who is the transcendent.

[30] Sermon 32.

religion. God is but an aspect, and that must mean but an appearance of the Absolute.'[31]

The two-fold process of cosmicisation in the Yogic transformation of human nature can clearly be observed in the example of the most famous form of Yoga, the *darśana* of Patañjali, with its traditional eight members (*aṣṭāṅga*). Before we proceed to give an enumeration and description of these divisions of the classical *yoga-mārga*, we would like to introduce a slightly modified representation of the stages of Pātañjalayoga. The sequence of stages given below is based on the second chapter (*pāda*) of Patañjali's text book. The reader himself, referring back to the Sanskrit original, will have to decide how far our reconstruction is justified.

I. *yama*
II. *niyama*

saṃtoṣa — *svādhyāya* — *tapas* — *īśvara-praṇidhāna* — *śauca*

(1) *āsana*
(2) *prāṇāyāma*
(3) *pratyāhāra*
(4) *dhāraṇā*
(5) *dhyāna*
(6) *samādhi*

Counter to this, the traditional scheme is:

yama — 'restraint', ethical precepts regulating the social life
niyama — 'observance', ethical precepts with regard to the inner life
āsana — 'seat' or bodily posture
prāṇāyāma — 'control of life energy'
pratyāhāra — 'withdrawal' of the senses from the outer world
dhāraṇā — 'binding' of the mind, usually translated by concentration
dhyāna — '[concentrated] reflection', commonly called meditation
samādhi — 'unification', best rendered as enstasis

Prior to embarking on a discussion of the specific character of each of these steps with regard to the operation of the cosmicisation, we need

[31] F. H. Bradley, *Appearance and Reality*, 10th impr. (London, Oxford University Press, 1969), p. 396–7

to outline the nature of the worldly man from the point of view of Yoga. The worldly man is a being who is in constant conflict with himself, the world, other beings and with—here lies the root of the whole dilemma—the transcendent reality. Perhaps it would not be going too far astray if we designate man as that entity who exists in a situation of most acute dichotomy and who possesses the capacity of realising this and actually freeing himself from this antagonistic condition. This basic discord in human nature was the subject of many of Blaise Pascal's aphorisms, one of which runs as follows:

> Inner war in man between reason and the passions. If there was only reason without passions. . . . If there were only the passions without reason. . . . But since both are, man cannot be without strife, for he can be at peace only with the one if he is at war with the other; that way he is always divided and in conflict with himself.[32]

Man is the dualistic being *par excellence*. He is, as Nietzsche harshly expressed it, a rope stretched between animal and God. We choose to slightly modify this metaphor and take man to be animal and God as well as the rope, whereby the rope is to symbolise the mind and its mediating function. It is the mind which makes man what he is, enabling him to be more brutish than any animal (as Mephistopheles is made to say in Goethe's *Faust*) and to be more divine than God (as Eckehart and the Indian yogins tried to convey). This has been fully understood by all adepts of Yoga, Eastern and Western, to whom the mind always was, as Evans-Wentz phrased it, the 'supreme magician'. In the *Amṛtabindu-Upaniṣad* it is stated:

> The mind (*manas*) is declared to be two-fold, pure and impure. The impure [mind] is desire-will (*kāma-saṃkalpa*), the pure [mind] is devoid of desire.
> The mind, indeed, is the cause of man's bondage and liberation. Attached to objects it is said to [lead] to bondage, [when] free of objects to liberation.[33]

In other words, it is the mind, illumined by the transcendent, that

[32] This translation is based on W. Weischedel's German rendering. The aphorism is number 412 in León Brunschwicg's edition of the *Pensées*, published Paris 1904.
[33] Stanzas 1–2. *Cf. Viṣṇu-Purāṇa* VI.7.28.

renders it possible to bring about the transformation of human nature. This is the central theme of Yoga, and, naturally, Yoga starts with an inventory of the psychomental contents. That is why Vyāsa, in his commentary to the *Yoga-Sūtra*, begins with a mention of the five levels of functioning of the mind which are: the 'unsteady' (*kṣipta*), the 'confused, muddy' (*mūḍha*), the 'distracted' (*vikṣipta*) the 'one-pointed' (*ekāgra*) and the 'restricted' (*niruddha*). The first three types of mental activity are common to what we earlier designated as the worldly man, the Sanskrit equivalent of which is *pṛthag-jana* which carries a far deeper philosophical meaning than generally supposed, for *pṛthak* signifies something which is 'apart': the worldly man is split off from the Absolute. This 'apartness' or isolation forms the radix of his relativity, impotence and consequent suffering (*duḥkha*). To the Indian sage the only heresy there can be is the heresy of separateness, from which stems all the evil of the world. It is characteristic of the Vedas, for example, that the oneness which is the hallmark of the spiritual life is subtly, but constantly, brought out, especially by means of such a grand figure as Agni, the all-pervading fire, which burns in all things, animate and inanimate. It is the growing consciousness of his historicity that holds in store so much pain for modern man, since the realisation of his own impermanence confronts him with death which, being bare of all religious meaning, can only signal such anguished prospects as annihilation and nothingness.[34] Applying Indian standards, we can say that the mind of the present-day worldly man is basically *mūḍha* or defiled by *tamas*, the power of inertia, which blinds, darkens, covers and draws away from the light of purer realms. Lacking even the minimum belief in a spiritual order beyond the material world, he is unable to cherish any conscious desire for something different from mundane objects and values. He chiefly moves within the two lowest spheres of human activity, sensual enjoyment and material achievement,[35] regarding morality only as 'useful' insofar as it promotes personal interests. The whole situation has time and again been circumscribed by one word: *kali-yuga*, the age of darkness, blasphemy and spiritual death. This is what we meant when, in the preface, we referred

[34] *Cf.* M. Eliade, *Myths, Dreams and Mysteries*, transl. by Philip Mairet (London and Glasgow, 1968), pp. 232f.

[35] Indian philosophy postulates four great aims of human life: sensual enjoyment (*kāma*), material achievement (*artha*), righteousness (*dharma*) and emancipation (*mokṣa*).

to the crisis of man, the world-crisis.[36] After this short excursion, we can return to our consideration of the Yogic path which professes to lead man from the chaos of the mundane life to a state in harmony with the cosmos and, then, even beyond it, into that realm beyond the sun where 'there is another glory', as one of the ancient Vedic sages put it poetically.[37] Naturally, this transmutation is a gradual process. Human personality cannot be radically changed from one moment to the next. This is why, in the scriptures of Yoga, steadiness (*dhṛti*), perseverance (*dhairya*), patience (*kṣamā*) and energy (*vīrya*) as well as Attic faith (*śraddhā*) are considered to be preliminary qualities of the student. The path is steep and studded with obstacles, and the goal is distant.

The first step towards it is to harmonise one's social relationships. This is done on the basis of a recognition of the fellow-man as being *essentially* of the same reality as oneself. This, in fact, is extended to all living beings and, in the higher stages of Yoga, even to the last particle of the universe, the living cosmos, as signified so appropriately by the Sanskrit work *jagat* (√ *gā* 'to go'), which, at its base, is non-different from the Absolute. Thus man is to transcend his own personality and to view the worldly affairs from an absolute standpoint. A beautiful example of this is given in the charming and highly esoteric *Īśa-Upaniṣad*:

> But he who beholds all beings in his own Self, and his own Self in all beings, does no longer hate (*vijugupsate*).[38]

We have indicated how this is possible when explaining the two-faced Janushead of the mind which is either directed towards the transpersonal reality or involved in the machinery of the empirical personality ruled by the animalic desires of the physical vehicle (*sthūla-śarīra*). Why the regulation of the social life should be the first to be attempted by the yogin is explained by the fact that in this sphere of human

[36] However, on account of a critical study of history, we venture to differ from the classical Indian conception of the *kali-yuga* insofar as we take this dark age as coming to an end at present. In this connection it is of significance to note that according to the Sanskrit texts themselves the traditional theory of the *yugas* has no universal validity, but is restricted to India. *Cf.* F. E. Pargiter, *Ancient Indian Historical Tradition* (London, Oxford University Press, 1922), pp. 175f. And also D. R. Mankad, 'The Yugas', *The Poona Orientalist*, VI (1941–2), pp. 206–16.

[37] *Ṛgveda* X.27.21.

[38] Stanza 6.

activity the coarsest violations against and infractions of the order (*ṛta*) inherent in the cosmos are perpetrated which, by the law of causation effective even on the ethical level (as *karma* and *karma-vipāka*), produce unwholesome results and bind man to the ever-turning wheel of existence (*bhava-cakra*). The whole field of social conduct is, in Yoga, covered by the various precepts of *yama* or 'restraint', the first *aṅga* of the Pātañjalayoga, with *śīla* as its Buddhist equivalent.[39] The *Yoga-Sūtra* (II.30) enumerates five rules under the heading of *yama*:

ahiṃsā	— 'non-harming', usually translated by non-violence, which encompasses not only physical action, but also thought and feeling
satya	— 'truth(fulness),' in speech and mind
asteya	— 'non-stealing'
brahmacarya	— chastity or sexual continence in action and thought
aparigraha	— 'greedlessness'

These have to be exercised without regard to social standing, location, time or circumstances and are, if mastered, also called the 'great vow' (*mahā-vrata*).[40] This ethical code is, with slight modifications, common property of almost all religions. Sometimes five more rules are mentioned in the Yoga texts:

dayā	— 'compassion'
ārjava	— 'straightforwardness'
kṣamā	— 'patience'
dhṛti	— 'steadiness'
mitāhāra	— 'temperance'

These can be taken as actually contained in the body of the first five rules. The purpose of these relentless demands is obvious. They try to replace negative volitions, emotions and habits, like hatred, verbosity or overacting, by positive and sound inner states founded upon the recognition that the individual is non-different from all other existing entities and that he can call nothing his 'own', wherefore he has to

[39] The Buddhist *pañca-śīla* and the Yogic *yama* differ from each other in one entry only. The last precept of the former set refers to slothfulness caused by drinks and drugs which, in the YS, is not mentioned. But this rule is not always included into the series, which is predicative of its secondary importance.
[40] *Vide* YS II.31.

eradicate all aforementioned negative actions, feelings and thoughts in order not to influence the fellow-beings in an unwholesome way. That even the propelling force behind physical deeds, the mind, from its own level, is able to affect the environment, is a fact Western man has not yet awakened to. This incontestable truth has, so far, only penetrated the minds of a small circle of adepts and a mere handful of more daring scientists who encountered it in the course of their experimental studies of certain mental phenomena such as telepathy and telekinesis, the latter being by far the greater puzzle of the two and being, accordingly, not yet fully recognised even by those who experimented with it. In Yoga, which is far more advanced in the study and application of the mind than any of the many branches of psychology, these so-called 'psychic' or, according to the modern scientific nomenclature, parapsychological phenomena are quite familiar sights. But, as already mentioned, they are not given much attention by the yogin who, having set his mind to win the highest goal still in this life, makes no use of them, unless it be to help another being and then, only after due consideration. These powers or, as they are termed in Yoga, *siddhis* or *vibhūtis*, are given a more eminent place in those forms of Yoga which are, like Haṭhayoga and the different offshoots of the Tantric *sādhana*, to a certain degree influenced by popular aims and ideals. And here again, it is highly indicative that, in the experience of Purohit Swāmi, the *haṭhayogins* 'have great powers, strong healthy bodies and immense vanity . . . They were generally amenable to praise, and some *more worldly than average worldly man.*'[41]

The second member (*aṅga*) of Yoga, according to the *Pātañjala-Sūtra*, aims at a harmonisation of the 'inner life' as opposed to social relationships. Though living in harmony with one's fellow-beings is imperative, this alone cannot bring about the desired Self realisation (*ātma-anubhava*), for man is not only what he is, but also what he was, that is, by the practice of *yama* the surface personality can be re-shaped, but the subconscious formative factors or *saṃskāras* remain untouched. The importance of this fact may best be grasped when we resort to the well-known graphic representation of the different levels of consciousness in form of an iceberg which is nine-tenths submerged and one-

[41] Shree Purohit Swāmi, *Aphorisms of Yoga*, 3rd ed. (London, 1957), p. 30. The book, a valuable popular introduction, was prefaced by W. B. Yeats. The italics are ours.

tenth visible. This comparison is of course only of a rather limited value, alone by reason of the fact that the personal subconscious, the part under water, is far too deep to justify any comparison with the waking consciousness. In fact, it must be limitless, since it, in unobservable degrees, goes over into the impersonal subconscious containing all the numberless traces left behind by the immeasurable number of beings who, in countless aeons, struggled in the universe for Self realisation. It is these *saṃskāras*, keeping in store the fruits of past deeds (*karma*), which the yogin is to root out completely, if he wants to gain the desired emancipation.

Niyama which we translate by 'observance' is, like *yama* made up of a number of rules. In the *Yoga-Sūtra* five such regulative principles are enumerated:[42]

śauca	— 'cleanliness' including inner purity
saṃtoṣa	— 'contentment'
tapas	— lit. 'fire', standing for ascetic exercises
svādhyāya	— lit. 'own going into', referring to study of the scriptures as well as to the repetition of certain formulas (*mantras*)
īśvara-praṇidhāna	— devotion to the 'lord'.

These require some explanation. *Śauca* covers every type of cleansing practice as well as the effort to abstain from impure thoughts and emotions and as such is a continuation of *brahmacarya*, the fourth rule of *yama*. The *Yoga-Bhāṣya* of Vyāsa states: 'Inner [purity] is the washing away of the impurities of the mind (*citta-mala*).'[43] *Saṃtoṣa* stands in connection with one of the central terms of the *Bhagavad-Gītā*; it is, in a sense, a branch of equanimity (*samatva*). *Samatva* is a positive value, for it not only creates an inner balance which enables the yogin to think and act calmly and appropriately, but it also gives rise to a centre of bliss within him which, when fully developed, will influence the environment sometimes to a remarkable degree.[44] Anyone who has

[42] *Vide* YS II.32.

[43] YBh. II.32.

[44] *Cf.* YS II.42: 'As a result of *saṃtoṣa* [there comes about] peerless happiness (*sukha*).' The importance of this practice is further stressed by the following statement of the BhG: 'Yoga is called equanimity' (*samatvaṃ yoga ucyate*. II.48).

sat at the feet of a yogin, advanced on the path, will be able to give testimony to this.

Early mention of the practice of *tapas* (ἄσκησις) can be found in the *Ṛgveda* where it holds a decisive position among those techniques which were later integrated into the Yogic path. Indeed, *tapas* may well be the oldest element of Yoga. It stood in close connection with the Vedic sacrifice, the *yajña*, where it performed the function of a preliminary exercise. Let us here take a brief look at the sacrifice itself which, together with the conceptions of *ṛta* and *satya*, forms the foundation of Vedic religious culture. The purpose of every sacrifice is after all to attract the attention of the hidden higher powers (*numina*) in the universe which, though invisible, nevertheless, according to our ancestors, play a dominant part in the success or failure of worldly affairs. The formalistic element of the sacrifice—*i.e.* the giving and returning of a gift—does not at all exhaust its function. Far more important is the mystical contact which is established between the sacrificer, the sacrificial gift and the hidden powers accepting it.[45] One section of the Vedic priests appears to have been particularly interested in this aspect of the sacrifice. They not only sacrificed for reasons of penance or supplication, but also in order to come into communication and, indeed, communion with the gods (*devas*), the rulers of the worlds beyond. This is supported by the fact that √ *yuj*, from which the term *yoga* is derived, is most frequently used in connection with the sacrifice, thus indicating a strict mental discipline underlying the *yajña*. J. W. Hauer, who was the first to trace the stream of Yogic ideas beyond the time of the Upaniṣads back to the Vedic period, made the following remark:

> It follows from the nature of the old Indian sacrifice that Yoga in the indicated sense [as original or *Uryoga*] was most intimately connected with it. He who is not able to yoke his thoughts, sacrifices ineffectively past the supernatural entity.[46]

[45] The highly esoteric character of the Vedic *yajña* is evident from the fact that a successful sacrifice presupposed a profound change in the sacrificer, his transformation into a 'superman' or *ati-mānuṣa*. Hence, according to the *Śatapatha-Brāhmaṇa* (I.1.16), he had to repeat the following words after the sacrificial act: 'Now I am [again] he who I really am.' With this magical formula he broke the power of the vow (*vrata*) and regained his human consciousness.

[46] J. W. Hauer, *Der Yoga. Ein indischer Weg zum Selbst*, p. 20.

Now, *tapas* was considered one of the accessories, perhaps even the most important one, to that state of concentration regarded as absolutely necessary for a correct and effective sacrificial act. The word is derived from $\sqrt{}$ *tap*, meaning 'to burn, heat', and covers such practices as fasting, standing erect and still in the burning sun, keeping absolute silence over a long period and bearing extreme heat or cold. These techniques, reminding one of certain coarse mortifications in *kuṇḍalinī-yoga*,[47] were designed to produce a 'psychic heat' which led to shiftings within the mental structure in the direction of a supra-consciousness serving as a base for visionary experiences, auditions, exaltations and ecstasies. Though this type of rigorous self-castigation was present in all phases of Yoga—even the Buddha pursued it for some time—there have always been some outstanding yogins who did not hesitate to regard this form of *tapas* as self-destructive and not inducive of the highest goal. Bhīṣma, the celebrated hero of the *Mahābhārata*, for example, declares:

> What people consider to be *tapas*, [like] fasting through half the month, is in fact only an impairment of the body and is, by good people, not regarded as *tapas*.
>
> Renunciation (*tyāga*) and humility are to be taught as the highest *tapas*; he who has got these two virtues, has also the continued fasting and persisting chastity.[48]

This is in conformity with the *Yoga-Sūtra*: 'Through *tapas* [comes about], after the impurity has dwindled, perfection of the body [and its] organs.'[49] Here is spoken of a perfection (*siddhi*) of the body, not of its mutilation and destruction.

The next subdivision of *niyama* is *svādhyāya*, made up of *sva* ('own')

[47] The main aim of this Yoga is to gain Self realisation by awakening and manipulating the 'serpent power', the immanent or energy (*śakti*) aspect of the transcendent reality as confined to the body. In the unawakened or ordinary person, *kuṇḍalinī* 'sleeps'—in the subtle body—at the base of the spine, mainly stimulating the reproductive organs. The yogin has raised this psychic force to the crown of the head where the *śakti* re-unites with the Śiva, the transcendent. This practice is said to lead to both emancipation (*mukti*) and enjoyment (*bhukti*).

[48] Mbh. XII.221.4–5. *Cf.* BhG XVII.5–6.

[49] YS I.43: *kāya-indriya-siddhir-aśuddhi-kṣayāt tapasaḥ*.

and *adhyāya* ('going into') and having the double meaning of '[one's] own study [of something]' or 'study of [one's] own'. In the first sense the word is commonly applied to the study of the holy scriptures (*śāstras*) or to the recitation of magical words (*mantras*). Its second connotation is more esoteric in nature; though still referring to the practice of studying the *śāstras* and reciting *mantras*, it stresses their effect on the mind of the individual. A passage from the *Śatapatha-Brāhmaṇa* may here serve as an illustration:

> The study and propounding [of the sacred scriptures] are [a source] of pleasure [to the serious student]. He becomes of subdued mind (*yukta-manas*) and independent of others, and day by day he acquires [spiritual] power. He sleeps peacefully, and he is the best physician (*cikitsaka*) for himself. [He possesses] restraint of the senses (*indriya-saṃyama*) [and has] delight in the One, growth of insight (*prajñā*) and [inner] glory (*yaśas*) [and the wish of] promoting the world.[50,51]

Last we have to consider *īśvara-praṇidhāna*, the fifth precept of the body of 'observations'. This rule was for long the subject of scholarly discussions and suffered a great deal of misinterpretation. These debates were called forth by the fact that in Pātañjalayoga the 'lord' or *īśvara* appears to hold a somewhat obscure position. For he is regarded as one of the multiple transcendent Selves (*puruṣas*) or soul-monads, and yet considered to be a special Self (*viśeṣa-puruṣa*), being eternally untouched by the causes of suffering (*kleśas*), action (*karma*) and its fruit (*vipāka*) as well as the subconscious depositions (*saṃskāras*).[52] In other words, he remains through all time a transcendent entity which never has been and never will be anything else but this, while all other Selves, at some stage or other, were or will be ensnared in the cycles of nature or *prakṛti*. In the opinion of a number of scholars this theological teaching shows grave inconsistencies and is incompatible with the dualistic standpoint of Patañjali. To them *īśvara* is an obtruder who, by the favour of some theistic redacteur of the *Yoga-Sūtra*, obtained his position quite surreptitiously. But *īśvara* did not enter Yoga from the

[50] The Sanskrit word *loka-pakti* literally means 'cooking of the world'.
[51] *Śatapatha-Brāhmaṇa* XI.5.7.1.
[52] YS: I.24: *kleśa-karma-vipāka-āśayair aparāmṛṣṭaḥ puruṣaviśeṣa īśvaraḥ*. The five *kleśas* are: ignorance (*avidyā*), 'I-am-ness' (*asmitā*), passion (*rāga*), aversion (*dveṣa*) and clinging to life (*abhiniveśa*). *Vide* YS II.3.

outside; he was from earliest times a principal feature of it.[53] We would even go so far as to assert that Hinduistic Yoga ends where the belief in God terminates. True, original Yoga always was and will be *sa-īśvara* or 'with God'.[54] For God is a reality which, according to the testimony of the yogins and mystics of different countries and ages, can be experienced. This was the only reason why Patañjali, in his compendium, included God at all. Unlike Kapila, the legendary founder of the Sāṃkhya system, he tried to formulate the position of *īśvara* within his dualistic system. But even if Patañjali had kept silent on this point, he would probably not have escaped the criticism of later 'interpreters', as can be seen by the example of the Buddha. Since Patañjali taught the dualism of matter and spirit, *prakṛti* and *puruṣa*, he naturally placed God in the latter category. This way *īśvara* became a *puruṣa*, one of the many Selves. So far Patañjali's teaching is in agreement with Advaita-Vedānta which likewise makes a distinction between the illusory[55] world and the transcendent *ātman*. This interpretation may be considered superficial by some who argue that according to classical Yoga there is a plurality of Selves while in Advaita-Vedānta there is One only, that Patañjali regarded the world as real while Śaṅkara saw it as a dream. However, to our mind, these are mere side-issues of no importance for the statement of the present problem. One has to bear in mind that qualitatively there is no difference between the Selves (*puruṣas*) of Patañjali and the one Self (*ātman*) of Śaṅkara. The diverse Indian soteriological systems (*mokṣa-śāstras*) unfortunately tend to be viewed by Western scholars from all possible angles, except from the one they set out to present. Thus there are but few who have fully recognised that all these *darśanas* or 'world-views' (in the widest possible sense) are axiological systems *per se*, their primary interest being the liberation of man and not psychological, ontological or existentialistic discussions.[56]

But to return to the precept of *īśvara-praṇidhāna*. God, though recog-

[53] This point of view is supported by the historical facts, as found in the Mbh., which were ably delineated by P. M. Modi, *Akṣara. A Forgotten Chapter in the History of Indian Philosophy*, Inaugural Dissertation (Baroda, 1932), pp. 81f.

[54] *Cf.* Mbh. XII.300.3: 'How can one be liberated without the lord?' (*anīśvaraḥ kathaṃ mucyate.*)

[55] Illusory, however, does not imply non-existence, as wrongly held by some critics of Vedānta.

[56] *Vide* R. P. Singh, *The Vedānta of Śaṅkara: A Metaphysics of Value*, vol. I (Jaipur, 1949).

nised as having reality, is said not to be given any prominent place in the *Yoga-Sūtra*, since he is neither the creator nor the container or destroyer of the world as is the case in the Semitic tradition. This view, resulting from the theory that *īśvara* came into the Pātañjalayoga by way of interpolation, is untenable. If our reconstruction of the path of the *Yoga-Sūtra* is correct,[57] *īśvara-praṇidhāna* is to be accepted as one of the five categories of Yoga practice proper, the other four being *tapas*, *svādhyāya*, *saṃtoṣa* and *śauca*. But even if our attempt is discarded, there are a number of aphorisms which unassailably demonstrate the importance of this practice. In the *Yoga-Sūtra* it is thus clearly affirmed: 'Or [restriction of the psychomental flux can be achieved] through devotion to the lord.'[58] To this Vyāsa makes the following comment: 'Through devotion (*praṇidhāna*), [which is] a special love (*bhakti-viśeṣa*), [the yogin wins the "sympathy" of the lord and] *īśvara* inclines [to him] favouring him on account of his deep devotion only.'[59] Furthermore, in the *Yoga-Sūtra* it is stated: 'Attainment of the enstasis (*samādhi*) [results] through devotion to the lord.'[60] Finally, one must also consider the aphorisms pertaining to the recitation of the *mantra* '*oṃ*' which is declared to be the symbol of the lord.[61]

Īśvara and *puruṣa*, like the Vedāntic *brahman* and *ātman*, are *essentially* non-different. This is borne out by the fact that both are considered to be omnipresent and omniscient. Two all-knowing or all-pervasive realities cannot exist apart from each other. As already stated, the transcendent 'situation', that is, the inner relationship between Self and God, is beyond human imagination and inexpressible. All descriptions are therefore partial truths only. When Patañjali conceives a certain difference between these two aspects of the Absolute, calling the *īśvara* a special *puruṣa*, he is correct, and at the same time, wrong. For according to the statements made by philosophically trained persons *with the experience of the transcendent reality*,[62] the manifold does not

[57] *Vide* p. 11.
[58] YS I.23: *īśvara-praṇidhānād-vā.*
[59] YBh. I.23.
[60] YS II.45: *samādhi-siddhir-īśvara-praṇidhānāt.*
[61] YS I.27–9: 'His symbol is the *praṇava* [*i.e. oṃ*]. Its meditative recitation [leads to] the realisation of its meaning. Thereupon [follows] the introversion of consciousness and also the removal of the [nine] obstacles.' (*tasya vācakaḥ praṇavah. taj-japas-tadartha-bhāvanam. tataḥ pratyak-cetanā-adhigamo'py-antarāya-bhāvaś-ca.*)
[62] It could be assumed that Patañjali's peculiar point of view is due to his never having had this experience, but there is no immediate reason for this conjec-

cease to exist in the Absolute, only the singularising human consciousness is abandoned. However, to view *īśvara* as something not absolutely identical with the Self is of intrinsic *practical* value. Not only does it enable souls of a more devotional constitution to advance on the path by way of *praṇidhāna* or 'devotedness', but also warns the yogin with a more intellectual outlook not to think of himself in terms too great, thus falling prey to dangerous pride (*abhimāna*). In monistic systems, like the Advaita-Vedānta, there is always the danger of purely intellectually identifying oneself with the Absolute before having realised the truth of *ahaṃ brahma-asmi*. In an adept not yet completely stabilised in the attitude of non-attachment or *vairāgya* this may easily lead away from the path. These practical considerations seem never to have occurred to the critics of Patañjali's system. Thus R. C. Zaehner makes the following unwise comment:

> God, in the classical Yoga, is nothing more than a *deus ex machina* invented for the purpose of explaining how the individual *puruṣas* ever became involved in *prakṛti*; and this appears to be his only function. It is perhaps the strangest conception of 'God' known to the whole of religion.[63]

The different constituents of *niyama*, especially *tapas*, lead over to the third stage of the Yogic path, namely *āsana* or 'posture' which, on account of the growing interest in Haṭhayoga, has become an almost familiar term in the West. It was shown how, by the rules of *yama* and *niyama*, the yogin takes the first measures for his liberation inasmuch as he regulates his life as a social being as well as an individual, thus avoiding the production of any further negative, unwholesome volitions or their physical expressions as deeds which only would involve him more in the conditioned existence or *saṃsāra*. His next step is to eradicate the impressions of his former thoughts and actions, the *saṃskāras*, left in his subconscious mind, which are harmful whether they were caused by wholesome volitions or not, because by their sheer presence they bind man unto the eternal rolling of cosmic existence. The yogin, striving for absolute freedom (*mokṣa*) or pure

ture. Instead it leaves out of consideration the fact that the author of the *Yoga-Sūtra* was, in all probability, also a recognised teacher of a particular school of Yoga and as such should have been skilled in the higher practices of Yoga.

[63] R. C. Zaehner, *Mysticism, Sacred and Profane* (Oxford, 1957), p. 127.

being-ness (*kaivalya*), must not only disarm but fully uproot them. The only means to do this is by delving into himself and sending the plummet of his concentrated mind right down into the abyss of his subconsciousness. This practice, however, can only be carried out in quiet surroundings and with the body put at rest so as to get the minimum amount of sense-impressions from outside and from within the physical vehicle. Thus *āsana* has the function of putting the body into a most relaxed position to assure the highest possible comfort.[64] That is what Patañjali meant when formulating: 'The posture [has to be] steady [and] comfortable.'[65] And to make the point quite clear, he adds: '[This] practice [is to be done] with relaxation [and] coinciding with Ananta.'[66] According to the explanations of Vācaspati Miśra, Ananta is here the mythical ruler of the serpents who holds the globe in balance, thus symbolising equilibrium in general and poise of mind in particular.[67] In the *Tejobindu-Upaniṣad* we can read:

> That in which constant reflection on *brahman*, the principle of all, is possible without effort is called *āsana*; any change in it destroys the experience of joy.[68]

Āsana is a good example of the fact that all Yogic practices are interconnected and one step penetrates the other, the main aim always being the concentration of the mind; even in the Gaṭhasthayoga, involving physical exercises only and as such the coarsest form of Haṭhayoga,[69] this end was not completely lost sight of. While the original purpose of *āsana* was to assist the meditative efforts of the yogin, this member of the Yogic path, in later developments, elaborated in great detail and given the additional function of serving as a means of strengthening the physical body for the strenuous mental exercises. This change was introduced by those following the Tantric path of transformation which,

[64] Symbolically, *āsana* is the imitation of a static and thus non-human reality. M. Eliade observes that it is, in a way, a one-pointedness (*ekāgratā*) on the physical level. *Vide* M. Eliade, *Yoga: Immortality and Freedom*, p. 54.

[65] YS II.46: *sthira-sukham-āsanam*.

[66] YS II.47: *prayatna-śaithilya-ananta-samāpattibhyām*. J. W. Hauer's reading is *anantya* (the 'endless') instead of *ananta* which, to us, seems more appropriate in this context.

[67] *Vide Tattva-Vaiśāradī* II.47.

[68] *Tejobindu-Up.* I.25.

[69] In the *Gheraṇḍa-Saṃhitā*, however, the term *gaṭhastha-yoga* is used as a synonym of *haṭhayoga*.

as a movement, originated some time in the first centuries A.D. But a number of different postures were already known in the time of the Buddha and still earlier. However, as the body was generally regarded as a burden and even hindrance to salvation in the pre-Christian era, it is unlikely that any experiments were made with regard to the physiological effect of certain postures;[70] this was seemingly the privilege of the *gurus* of Haṭhayoga, like Matsyendra, Gorakṣa or Gheraṇḍa, who, in their works, vividly describe the results that can be obtained from the execution of such practices. The reader interested in further studies on this feature of Yoga may refer to the excellent books by Theos Bernard, Alain Danielou and, of course, to the translations of the classical Sanskrit texts such as *Haṭhayoga-Pradīpikā*, *Gheraṇḍa-Saṃhitā* and *Śiva-Saṃhitā*.[71]

Āsana already having led to a certain state of relaxation and calmness, the next stage, *prāṇāyāma*, has an even more decided effect upon the psyche of the practitioner. This is clearly substantiated by the term *prāṇāyāma* itself, for *prāṇa*, usually and insufficiently translated by 'breath', has reference to what, in the language of the Upaniṣads, is called the *prāṇamaya-kośa* or 'sheath formed of life energy', that is the *sūkṣma-śarīra* or 'subtle body' of later Yoga. *Prāṇāyāma* (*prāṇa* + *āyāma*) is thus the 'control of *prāṇa*', of which the regulation of breath is but the most external aspect. *Prāṇa* itself is derived from the prefix *pra* ('on, forth') and √*an* ('to breathe') and denotes 'vital energy, life' and as such is not unlike Bergson's *élan vital*. In the *Yoga-Sūtra* and its commentaries we do not find it explicitly expressed that *prāṇa* is not mere breath. This omission can be excused in the aphorisms themselves, but not in the two standard expositions by Vyāsa and Vācaspati Miśra. But this is only too characteristic of the native commentaries. While endlessly discussing matters of obviously secondary value only, they remain silent on topics of such great significance. For an expressive explanation of the nature of *prāṇa*, we must therefore turn to those

70 Typical for this negative attitude are the outpourings of the author of the *Maitrāyaṇīya-Upaniṣad* (I.3): '. . . in this ill-smelling, unsubstantial body, which is a conglomerate of bone, skin, muscle, marrow, flesh, semen, blood, mucus . . . what is the good of enjoyment of desires?' (Radhakrishnan's translation.)

71 *Vide* Th. Bernard, *Hathayoga: The Report of a Personal Experience* (London, 1950); A. Danielou, *Yoga: Method of Re-Integration* (London, 1949). The three Sanskrit works were published in the series Sacred Books of the Hindus (Allahabad, 1915).

scriptures of Yoga which stand in the tradition of Vedānta. Thus in the *Yoga-Vāsiṣṭha* (III.13.31), an enormous and fascinating work consisting of more than twenty-four thousand stanzas, the word *vāyu* being a synonym of *prāṇa* is defined as 'that which vibrates' (*spandate yat sa tad*). *Prāṇa* is *spanda-śakti* or the subtle 'vibratory power' penetrating the whole cosmos and every living being and even able to exercise influence on the mind (*citta*). In fact, the relation between *prāṇa* and *citta* life, energy and mind, is a very intimate one. And it is the discovery of this circumstance which led to the 'invention' of the *prāṇāyāma* and its ample elaboration particularly in Haṭhayoga. The importance attached to this exercise in the Haṭhayogic school can best be demonstrated by the fact that the *Gheraṇḍa-Saṃhitā* dedicates one whole chapter with ninety-six stanzas to *prāṇāyāma*, but forty-five stanzas only to *dhyāna* and *samādhi*. *Prāṇa* is the cosmic breath, the rhythmic oscillation effective on all levels of conditioned existence. Man, in the course of his evolution, has moved away from this original rhythm of the universe and became 'out of tune'. The cosmicisation or imitation of the cosmos, mentioned in the beginning of this essay, is nowhere more distinguishable than in the technique of *prāṇāyāma* which endeavours to restore the primeval rhythm and cosmic harmony as manifested in man, the microcosm. The rhythmisation of breath (which, in the end, is also a unification) is considered to be the most effective method of inducing the re-establishment of the harmony of the microcosm as an exact replica of the all-harmonious macrocosm. Breath and psyche are deeply interconnected. Though being neglected in modern medicine and psychology, this fact has been recognised in both India and Greece.[72] The rhythm of *prāṇa* is comparable to the ebb and flow of tidal waves, these two phases being designated as *prāṇa* and *apāna* respectively. Later, in connection with the human body, more detailed classifications of the great *prāṇa* stream were made, but they are subsidiary to the two cyclic movements of the cosmic vibratory energy. Usually, five such subdivisions of *prāṇa* are mentioned, namely *prāṇa*, *samāna*, *apāna*, *udāna* and *vyāna*. These are connected with certain functions and distributed over certain regions of the body.[73] In the

[72] In Greek the verb ψύχειν, from which is derived our psyche, means 'to breathe, respire', and in Sanskrit the word *ātman*, now generally applied to the innermost being, the Self, originally meant 'breath' as well; this, for example, can be made out in Ṛgv. X.16.3.

[73] These details are dealt with in Vyāsa's commentary (III.39): '*Prāṇa* has its

Yoga-Sūtra only *udāna* (III.39), *samāna* (III.40) and *prāṇa* (I.34), in its general sense, are named. But then we find an exact description of the technique of *prāṇāyāma* which, according to Patañjali, consists of four stages: out-breathing (*bāhya*), in-breathing (*abhyantara*), holding of breath (*stambha*) and finally what we term the 'inner breathing' manifesting itself in extreme concentration. In most Yoga texts the first three movements (Patañjali calls them *vṛttis*) bear the names *recaka*, *puraka* and *kumbhaka* respectively. We are most interested here in the 'inner breathing' which, in the *Yoga-Sūtra*, is simply referred to as the 'fourth' (*caturtha*).[74] This type of breathing must not be confused with the *kevala-kumbhaka* of Haṭhayoga which is nothing but an extreme form of *stambha-vṛtti*, the third movement of breathing, the suspension of breath over an unusually long period of time. As opposed to this, Patañjali's 'fourth' rhythm occurs involuntarily in deep concentration. In enstasis (*samādhi*) breathing can even fade away completely for many hours. The body then falls into a state of cataleptic rigidity being a poor expression of the richness of experience and fulness of the life within. The yogin has now pierced the tight fetters of the earthbound mechanism of the physical brain, and with widened and intensified consciousness he penetrates into the 'spiritual' dimension of the cosmos. But this is part of the last stage of the Yogic path, and after *prāṇāyāma* there still remain further stages to be traversed in order to reach *samādhi*, the entrance to the second phase of the process of cosmicisation.

The rhythmisation of breath as an imitation of the cyclic vibration of the cosmic *prāṇa*, the workings of which can be detected in such natural rhythms as high and low tide, day and night, menstruation, periodic pulsation of stars and so on, leads to profound changes within the mind, which in turn prepare the ground for the higher forms of concentration. *Prāṇāyāma* proper is performed with supreme attention which, in itself, leads to that focussing of awareness (*ekāgratā*) aimed at by the yogin. Again, we see that the control of the vital energy by way of breathing, like also *āsana*, is not merely a physical exercise, but is accompanied by certain psychomental phenomena. In other words,

course through the mouth and nose and its fluctuation extends as far as the heart. And *samāna*, since it distributes equally, has its fluctuation from the navel. *Apāna*, since it leads down, has its fluctuation as far as the sole of the foot. *Udāna*, since it leads up, has its fluctuation as far as the head. *Vyāna* is pervading. Among these *prāṇa* is predominant.' (J. H. Wood's translation.)

[74] *Vide* YS II.49–53.

all techniques falling under the headings of *āsana* and *prāṇāyāma* as, for example, the *mudrās* and *bandhas* of Haṭhayoga, are *psychosomatic* exercises. This point, unfortunately, is little understood by Western practitioners, some of whom, for instance, advocate—and to their own harm—enthusiastically demonstrate that the eighty-four classical postures of the Haṭhayogic school can be 'run off' in an hour or even less, that *prāṇāyāma* can be executed without regard to time, climate and personal morals; that the intricate blockings of the *prāṇa* by *mudrās* and *bandhas* can be done by any one and without the purificatory exercises prescribed in the Sanskrit works. A quotation from Shree Purohit Swāmi's commentary to the *Yoga-Sūtra* will stress this: 'People forget that Yama and Niyama form the foundation, and unless it is firmly laid, they should not practise postures and breathing exercises. In India and Europe, I came across some three hundred people who suffered permanently from wrong practices, the doctors on examination found that there was nothing organically wrong and consequently could not prescribe.'[75]

The next step of the Yogic *mārga* or path is *pratyāhāra*, the withdrawal of the senses from the objects of the outer world, a process often compared to a tortoise withdrawing its limbs.[76] The word itself is made up of the prefixes *prati* and *ā* and $\sqrt{}$*hṛ* meaning 'to hold, fetch'. It thus stands for the 'non-grasping' of sense-objects. Perhaps it is not inappropriate here to quote the great hero of the Advaita-Vedāntic camp, Śaṅkara Ācārya:

> The sense-objects (*viṣayas*) are even more venomous than the poison of a black snake. Poison kills one who takes it, but these [sense-objects] [destroy] one who merely looks at them with his eyes.[77]

The author of the *Viṣṇu-Purāṇa* therefore asserts that 'no yogin can accomplish Yoga without controlling his senses'.[78] There is some element of *pratyāhāra* in all stages, even in *āsana* (as is verified by *sūtra* II.48); it even exists on the ethical scale in form of *vairāgya* or dispassion which is the expression of a radical enquiry into the nature of

[75] Shree Purohit Swāmi, *Aphorisms of Yoga*, pp. 56–7.
[76] *Vide* BhG. II.58.
[77] *Viveka-Cūḍāmaṇi* 77.
[78] *Viṣṇu-Purāṇa* VI.7.44: *indriyāṇām-avaśyastair-na yogī yoga-sādhakaḥ.*

mundane objects and values and embraces a whole philosophy. However, active *pratyāhāra* follows in the classical Yoga after *prāṇāyāma.*

Patañjali simply states: 'The withdrawal [of the senses] is as it were the imitation of the nature of the mind by the senses by means of not connecting with their objects.'[79] And: 'Thence [results] supreme subjugation of the senses.'[80] Vyāsa, the author of the oldest extant commentary to the aphorisms, though not giving any practical counsel, makes an informative statement: 'Just as when the honey-maker-king [*madhukara-rāja i.e.* the queen-bee] flies up, the bees fly after [him], and when he settles down, they settle down after [him]—so when the mind (*citta*) is restricted, the sense-organs are restricted.'[81] This is a clear allusion to the intimate relation between the withdrawal of the senses and the technique of concentration (*dhāraṇā*), the next *aṅga* of the eight-fold path. The senses (*indriyas*) are sometimes compared to horses which are vicious and unruly when the reins, symbolising the analytical mind (*manas*), are not held firm, that is, when the mind is 'unyoked' (*ayukta*).[82]

The full implications of this supreme mastery (*paramā vaśyatā*) of the sense-organs, deriving from the perfected withdrawal of the senses, have not been depicted in the commentaries, for *pratyāhāra* not only leads to a subjugation of one's own senses, but by the power of *pratyāhāra* one also gains control over the sensory functions of others. Though not being of any importance for the Yogic transmutation itself, this ability explains such 'objective hallucinations' as the famous rope-trick which, as the German scholar L. Staudenmaier, theologist and professor of chemistry, has set forth, is based on the possibility of reversing the perceptual processes.[83]

The *aṣṭāṅgayoga* of Patañjali is traditionally divided into two sets of techniques, the one group being designated as 'outer members' (*bahir-aṅgas*), the other as 'inner members' (*antar-aṅgas*). All stages of the Yogic path treated so far belong to the former set. Concentration (*dhāraṇā*) is

[79] YS II.54: *sva-viṣaya-asaṃprayoge cittasya svarūpa-anukāra-iva indriyāṇāṃ pratyāhāraḥ.*

[80] YS II.55: *tataḥ paramā vaśyatā indriyāṇām.*

[81] YBh. II.54.

[82] *Vide Kaṭha-Up.* III.3–6.

[83] *Vide* L. Staudenmaier, *Die Magie als experimentelle Naturwissenschaft* (Leipzig, 1912).

the first 'inner member'. The *raison d'être* of this two-fold distinction is obvious. While the 'outer members' are, strictly speaking, preliminary exercises only, the 'inner members' constitute the actual path of transformation, by the agency of which the mind powerfully 'inclines towards liberation' (*kaivalya-prāgbhāra*). For however long a yogin may employ himself in the observation of ethical precepts, the practice of posture, the control of the vital energy and the withdrawal of the senses, if he wishes to win Self-realisation he must nevertheless gain complete mastery over his mind, the great architect of all one's sorrow and glory. With the practice of concentration the yogin takes the most decisive step on the path. It is the three final techniques of Yoga—*dhāraṇā*, *dhyāna* and *samādhi*—which lead to fundamental changes within the psychomental constitution of the adept or *sādhaka*, gradually liberating him from his self-imposed limitations as human being and transforming him into a transpersonal entity or *siddha*.

The word *dhāraṇā* is derived from √*dhṛ* ('to hold tight') and complemented by the suffixes *an* and *ā*; it has the meaning of 'binding, holding' and stands for the fixation (con-*centr*-ation) of the mind. The author of the *Triśikhi-Brāhmaṇa-Upaniṣad*, a later treatise expounding the eight-fold Yoga in the light of Vedānta, declares: 'Know concentration to be the holding of the mind in a motionless state.'[84] This is modelled on Patañjali's aphorism: 'Concentration is the binding of the mind to [one] place.'[85] Turning to Vyāsa's *Yoga-Bhāṣya*, we are told what this 'place' or 'point' (*deśa*) can be:

> Concentration is the binding of the mind as a [gross] fluctuation (*vṛtti*) only, to the navel-centre (*nābhi-cakra*), the lotus of the heart (*hṛdaya-puṇḍarīka*), the light in the head (*mūrdha-jyotis*), the tip of the nose (*nāsikāgra*), the tip of the tongue (*jihvāgra*) or to other places like this or to an external object.[86]

In his gloss *Tattva-Vaiśāradī*, Vācaspati Miśra completes these explanations:

> To this there is also a [saying from a] *Purāṇa*: 'Having mastered the vital energy (*pavana*) by way of *prāṇāyāma* and the sense-organs by

[84] *Triśikhi-Brāhmaṇa-Up.* 31: *cittasya niścalī-bhāvo dhāraṇā dhāraṇaṃ vidhuḥ.*
[85] YS III.1: *deśa-bandhaś-cittasya dhāraṇā.*
[86] YBh. III.1.

> way of withdrawal, he should make the mind rest upon an appropriate support (*śubha-āśraya*).'[87] Appropriate supports are external [objects] [such as] Hiraṇyagarbha, Vāsava, Prajāpati and so on.[88]

Concentration is sometimes identified with 'one-pointedness' (*ekāgratā*), but this is not quite correct, for the latter simply represents the arrest of the psychomental flow, while concentration implies a fixation of the mind in order to gain understanding; as such *dhāraṇā* is a creative act based on the principle of centralisation of consciousness.

Concentration must become a habit, part of the yogin's life, to bring full success. In the *Visuddhi-Magga* of Buddhaghoṣa mention is made of a story which illustrates this point. One day a beautiful young woman who ran away from her husband passed Mātissa, a Buddhist monk, who practised the contemplation of a skeleton (a way of developing aversion to physical beauty and detachment from worldly joys). She tried to get his attention by laughing loudly and tempting. Mātissa, surprised by this disturbance, looked up and his view fell on the shining teeth of the young woman. Immediately he associated this picture in his mind with the image of a skeleton, the object of his meditations. And when afterwards the monk met the husband searching for his wife, the only thing Mātissa could remember was:

> I know not who passed by,
> A man or a woman.
> What I saw—a skeleton,
> Bones linked up with bones.[89]

The fruit of successful concentration is meditation or *dhyāna*, the last member but one of the eight-fold Yoga. However, the practice of concentration is not fool-proof as is indicated, by a verse of the *Mahābhārata*: 'Unsuccessful concentrations, o friend, lead people on bad paths, like ships on the ocean without guides, o prince.'[90] The function of *dhyāna* (√ *dhyai*, 'to contemplate') is described in the *Yoga-Sūtra* thus: 'Meditation is the focussedness of *pratyayas* therein

[87] *Viṣṇu-Purāṇa* VI.7.45.
[88] TV III.1.
[89] *Visuddhi-Magga* I, pp. 20–1. Mentioned in S. K. Mukherjee, 'An Outline of Principal Methods of Meditation', *Visva-Bharati Annals*, vol. III (Santiniketan, 1950), pp. 122–3.
[90] Mbh. XII.302.55.

[*i.e.* in concentration].'[91] Without elucidating the much debated term *pratyaya*, this definition remains somewhat obscure. In the commentaries and sub-commentaries the word is used either in the sense of 'cause' or of 'knowledge, consciousness of something'. In the *Yoga-Sūtra* this term is employed in a technical sense, like so many other words hitherto considered to be vague and non-technical. This fact, not having been recognised so far, led to the common notion that the Yoga of Patañjali is merely a (badly done, as is often implied) compilation being grafted upon the Sāṃkhya philosophy, while the *Yoga-Sūtra*, quite to the contrary, is a highly original contribution towards a phenomenology of meditative consciousness, to which a critical examination of its contents will bear witness. Be this point accepted, it becomes self-evident that Patañjali should have used certain technical terms to mark some of the more distinct phenomena encountered during the process of Yogic involution.

Pratyaya, which may conveniently be translated by 'awareness', has frequently been identified with *vṛtti* or 'fluctuation'. This usage is incorrect, since both terms do signify two different things. It is true that wherever there is a *vṛtti* there is also a *pratyaya*, but the presence of a *pratyaya* does not always indicate a simultaneous occurrence of a fluctuation, the reason for this being the existing difference between the five classes of gross fluctuation (*citta-vṛttis*) and those supraconscious processes which Patañjali styles *vitarka*, *vicāra* and so on. *Pratyaya* is thus the generic term of *vṛtti* and *paravṛtti*, the latter word standing for the metaphysical insights (*prajñā*) gained in the enstasis connected with consciousness.

The purpose of meditation is to eliminate the gross fluctuations by way of focussing the ideational contents of consciousness or *pratyayas* on a common centre, held by the power of concentration. In practice there is no sharp distinction between concentration and meditation; the one is entering into the other by imperceptible degrees. It must be borne in mind that none of these *pratyayas* present in meditation are real acts of volition. They are merely passive internal perceptions and not, as R. Prasāda translated the word, 'mental efforts'.[92] In meditation every deliberately procured thought is experienced as a disturbance which, when strong enough, may lead to an abrupt end of the medita-

[91] YS III.2: *tatra pratyaya-ekatānatā dhyānam.*

[92] R. Prasāda, *Patanjali's Yoga Sutras*, Sacred Books of the Hindus, ed. by Major B. D. Basu, vol. IV (Allahabad, 1912).

tive disposition of the mind. However, thoughts of the nature of acts of volition or *vṛttis* are very frequent at the outset of meditation, and they play an important role in imagination exercises which are employed particularly in Tantrism. The mechanism of *dhyāna* is extremely intricate and still requires a thorough study.[93] Basically, it is a unification of the cognitive and affective elements of consciousness. It prepares for the enstatic experience. A specific type of meditation is employed in Haṭhayoga, where a distinction is made between coarse (*sthūla*), luminous (*jyotis*) and subtle (*sūkṣma*) meditation. Yogin Gheraṇḍa gives a descrition of these three forms which are complex and highly complicated imagination and visualisation exercises typical of Tantrism, one of which we subjoin:

> Let [the yogin] imagine that there is a great sea of nectar in his own heart; that in the middle of that [sea] there is an island of precious stones, the sand of which is pulverised gems; that on all sides of it are *nīpa*-trees laden with sweet flowers; that next to these trees, like a rampart, there is a row of flowering trees such as *mālatī*, *mallikā*. *jātī*, *kesara*, *campaka*, *pārijāta* and *padma*, and that the fragrance of these flowers is spreading all round in every quarter. In the middle of this garden, let the yogin imagine that there rises a beautiful *kalpa*-tree with four branches, representing the four Vedas, and that it is laden with flowers and fruits. Beetles are humming there and cuckoos are singing. Beneath that [tree] let him imagine a great platform of precious gems. Let the yogin imagine that in its middle there is a beautiful throne inlaid with jewels. On that [throne] let the yogin imagine his particular deity (*devatā*) as taught by the teacher [who will instruct him as to] the appropriate form, adornment and vehicle of that deity. Such a form constantly meditated upon—know this to be *sthūla-dhyāna*.[94]

It is obvious that this type of meditation is not suitable for a novice not yet endowed with the necessary power of concentration to produce such a rich imagery. He has to simply cast his full attention on one single point, like the space between the eyebrows or the rhythmic

[93] Some important psychological cum-phenomenological contributions to the study of the meditative consciousness have already been made. We would like to draw special attention to C. Albrecht, *Psychologie des mystischen Bewusstseins* (Bremen, 1951) and F. Heiler, *Die buddhistische Versenkung* (München, 1922).
[94] *Gheraṇḍa-Saṃhitā* VI.2–8.

beating of his heart. The advanced student can practise *trāṭaka* (relaxed gazing) on the flame of a candle and then close his eyes and concentrate on the after-image of the light. This is one form of *jyotir-* or *tejo-dhyāna*. An instructive account of this exercise and its effects is given by Theos Bernard who learned the technique from an Indian yogin and had success with it after two months of training.[95]

The last member and the consummation of the Yogic path of transmutation is *samādhi*. The importance of this stage is expressed by the preliminary definition of Yoga as given in the *Yoga-Bhāṣya*: 'Yoga is *samādhi*'.[96] It is from this technique that the arguments of Yoga derive their strength and value. Just as concentration, by appropriate depth and intensity, passes into meditation, so meditation gives place to the enstatic consciousness when the inner world (*citta*) has reached absolute calm (*nirodha*). The yogin then takes the last step to outstrip his human limitations, to change his very nature by transforming his empirical consciousness into a supramental consciousness. This is the final phase of the long process of de-humanisation which commenced with the refusal to move (in *āsana*), to breathe (in *prāṇāyāma*) and to engage in discursive thought (in *ekāgratā*). After the mind has become a *tabula rasa* by inhibiting the whirls (*vṛttis*) or activities of empirical consciousness in meditation, *samādhi* ensues.

The exact nature of this transpersonal 'experience' cannot be communicated, and this is probably the main reason for the unjust treatment it is constantly given by Western critics. As C. G. Jung noticed, to many *samādhi* is nothing but a 'meaningless dreamstate'.[97] The enstatic consciousness has been subject to a great amount of misunderstanding and misrepresentation. But, as Tagore observed, 'there is none who has the right to contradict this belief [*i.e.* the possibility of such supraconscious states]; for it is a matter of direct experience and not of logic'.[98] To fully understand the nature of *samādhi*, one must resort to personal experience. 'Yoga can [only] be known by Yoga', says Vyāsa.

[95] *Vide* Theos Bernard, *Hathayoga* pp. 75*ff*.

[96] YBh.I. 1: *yogaḥ samādhiḥ*.

[97] *Vide* C. G. Jung's psychological commentary to W. Y. Evans-Wentz, *The Tibetan Book of the Great Liberation* (London, Oxford University Press, 1954), p. xlviii.

[98] R. Tagore, *The Religion of Man*, Unwin Books (London, 1961), p. 128. *Cf.* YS I.49.

The enstatic experience evades definition. Hence circumscriptions must suffice. One of the clearest quasidefinitions is given by Patañjali: 'This same [*i.e.* meditation, *dhyāna*] [when] the object only is shining forth [in it] [and when the mind] is, as it were, empty of its own nature [which is its distinguishing between subject and object]—[this] is enstasis.'[99] These few words lay bare the basic function of the enstatic consciousness which is a total unification in which subject and object, perceiver and perceived, and the process of cognition melt together into one single act, and all opposites are lifted (*coincidentia oppositorum*). Then the mind is transcended and the thing, as it really is (*yathābhūta*), is known.

It is self-evident after these explanations that *samādhi* cannot be equated to trance if by this is meant a state of lessened awareness. Ramana Maharshi, the sage of Tiruvannamalai, employed a paradox to express this fact; he said that *samādhi* is 'sleep in the waking state' (*jāgrat-suṣupti*). This supramental realisation can also not be characterised as 'ecstasy', even though this is frequently done. Ecstasy being of the nature of an emotional exaltation is the cardinal technique of Shamanism, but it cannot be related to the tranquil, disciplined and systematic conscious involution of Yoga. We have therefore accepted M. Eliade's rendering of the word as *enstasis* or unification. The Swedish scholar S. Lindquist has tried to prove that Yoga is based entirely on principles of hypnosis and autosuggestion, but this thesis has no support and is contrary to the statements made in the Sanskrit texts which clearly distinguish between enstatic and hypnotic states of consciousness.[100] A more recent attempt in this fallacious direction is D. Langen's book.[101]

There are numerous modalities of this enstatic consciousness, a fact which renders an adequate representation and evaluation even more difficult. Depending on method and aim, the states of *samādhi* can differ greatly from one another. Thus there is an obvious distinction between the enstasis as realised in Vedānta, Tantrism, Buddhism[102] and classical Yoga. In the following sections we shall outline the diverse

[99] YS III.3: *tad-eva-artha-mātra-nirbhāsaṃ svarūpa-śūnyam-iva samāhdiḥ*. Vyāsa and the other classical commentators interpret this aphorism in a slightly different and, it seems, less coherent way.

[100] *Vide* S. Lindquist, *Die Methoden des Yoga* (Lund, 1932).

[101] *Vide* D. Langen, *Archaische Ekstase und asiatische Meditation* (Stuttgart, 1963).

[102] In Buddhism *samādhi* may simply mean one-pointedness or concentration. In its deepest sense, however, it is identified with *jhāna* (Pāli) of which eight grades are generally supposed to exist, namely four *rūpa-jhānas* and four *arūpa-jhānas*.

grades or stages of *samādhi* as taught by the author of the *Yoga-Sūtra* who was not only a compiler, as commonly thought, but a gifted philosopher as well. In the past, Patañjali's efforts were readily belittled, and preconceived notions and lack of real interest prevented a true appreciation of his work which contains a highly original contribution towards a critical phenomenology of enstatic states. The inconsistencies supposed to exist in his manual are easily resolved by an unbiassed examination and critical analysis of its contents.

Patañjali classifies the states of *samādhi* according to the nature of their accompanying awarenesses (*pratyayas*), that is, the contents of the respective supraconsciousness. He distinguishes between two classes of *samādhi*, the first covering all those enstatic states connected with supramental cognition (*prajñā*), the latter being devoid of any objective substratum and thus also transcending *prajñā*. The former category, also designated as the extrovertive type of enstasis, bears the designation of *saṃprajñāta-samādhi* or enstasis with supramental cognition and is subdivided into four types:

1. *vitarka-samādhi* (directed towards a gross object)
2. *vicāra-samādhi* (directed towards a subtle object)
3. *ānanda-samādhi* (enstasis connected with joy)
4. *asmitā-samādhi* (enstasis connected with 'I-am-ness')

The second class, the introvertive type of enstasis, may be divided into two phases:

1. *asaṃprajñāta-samādhi* (enstasis devoid of cognition)
2. *dharma-megha-samādhi* (the final stage before liberation)

The means to achieve any of the various degrees of *samādhi* are practice (*abhyāsa*), the positive aspect (*pravṛtti*) of the path, and renunciation (*vairāgya*), the negative aspect (*nivṛtti*).[103] The former consists of the techniques as presented in the first seven stages of the Yogic *mārga* which need to be executed with care and persistence.[104] Renunciation is passionlessness towards worldly and, as is expressly stated, heavenly

[103] *Vide* YS I.12: 'The restriction of these [fluctuations of the mind] [is achieved by] practice and renunciation.' (*abhyāsa-vairāgyābhyāṃ tan-nirodhaḥ.*)
[104] *Vide* YS I.13–14: 'Practice is here the effort in steadying [the mind].—But this [practice] [gains] "firm ground" [only] when cultivated for a long time, uninterruptedly [and] with proper attention.' (*tatra sthitau yatno'bhyāsah.—sa tu dīrgha-kāla-nairantarya-satkāra-āsevito dṛḍha-bhūmiḥ.*)

objects.[105] The respective function of these two means (*upāyas*), which have as their Western counterparts the *via negativa* and *via illuminativa*, is beautifully described in the *Yoga-Bhāṣya*:

> The stream of the mind (*citta-nadī*) flows both ways; it flows to the good, and it flows to the bad. The one commencing with discrimination (*viveka*) and ending in emancipation (*kaivalya*)—that is the stream to the good (*kālyaṇa*). The one commencing with non-discrimination (*aviveka*) and ending in conditioned existence (*saṃsāra*)—that is the stream to the bad (*pāpa*). Through renunciation (*vairāgya*) the flowing in direction to the worldly objects (*viṣayas*) is checked, and through the practice (*abhyāsa*) of discriminative vision (*viveka-darśana*) the stream of discrimination is laid bare. Thus the subjection (*nirodha*) of the psychomental flux is dependent upon both disciplines.[106]

When the fluctuations (*vṛttis*) of the mind have been restricted by way of a radical application of *abhyāsa* and *vairāgya*, the natural barriers between mind and object break down and both coincide. This process is elucidated by Patañjali as follows: 'With the cessation of the [psychomental] movements [*i.e.* with the becoming of the mind] like a precious gem [which takes on the colour of its resting place], [there comes about] a fusion (*samāpatti*) [with reference to either] the "perceiver", "perception" [or] the "perceived" [according to whether the mind] is resting on [one] of these [or] is coloured by [one] of these.'[107] This signifies that the subject breaks into the sphere of the object, fuses with it and reveals its innermost essence. Vācaspati Miśra formulates this thus: 'The experiencing [lit. 'enjoying', *ābhoga*] [of the object of concentration] is supramental cognition (*prajñā*) by an immediate apprehension (*sākṣātkāra*) of the true form [of the object].'[108] The 'true form' (*sva-rūpa*) is nothing else but the thing-in-itself which to Kant was unrecognisable. In *samādhi* the division

[105] *Vide* YS I.15: 'Renunciation is the consciousness of being master [on the part of a yogin] who is free from thirst for objects seen [or] revealed [in the scriptures].' (*dṛṣṭa-anuśravika-viṣaya-vitṛṣṇasya vaśīkāra-saṃjñā vairāgya.*)

[106] YBh. I.12.

[107] YS I.41: *kṣiṇa-vṛtter-abhijātasya-iva maṇer-grahitṛ-grahaṇa-grahyeṣu tat-stha-tad-añjanatā samāpattiḥ.* √*grah* actually means 'to grasp'. The 'grasper' is of course the Self.

[108] TV I.17.

between I (*aham*) and This (*idam*) disappears, thus making truthful cognition possible. The yogin gains the power of penetrating with his vision through the veil of the phenomenal world, the realm of name and form (*nāma-rūpa*), and to behold the heart of the object supporting his meditation. This cognition by identification can be carried out on different levels, because the object itself is compounded of several 'layers', that is, it exists on diverse strata of existence. It consists of a gross (*sthūla*) and a subtle (*sūkṣma*) aspect, the latter having again multiple strata.

According to Yoga metaphysics the empirical cosmos is but the outer aspect of a vast universe, the true depth of which can only be fathomed by meditation. Our physical eyes perceive a three-dimensional universe only. Its spiritual depth is beyond the range of the normal human vision which works, even when aided by technical devices, on a very limited scale. Only the rays of the 'divine eye' (*divya cakṣus*), the *acies mentis* of St. Augustine, *i.e.* the unified consciousness, can penetrate into this hidden dimension of the world and reveal its mysterious workings, a glimpse of which the ordinary clairvoyant may catch simply by way of a special disposition. His vision, however, reaches not further than the first level of the subtle reality, usually called the 'astral' realm, a term which is vague and misleading. Patañjali uses his own nomenclature. He terms the different 'layers' of the cosmos (*prakṛti*) in the following way:

I Non-Manifest or transcendent principle of nature (*aliṅga*)
II Manifested world
  a) *liṅga-mātra* = *mahān* or *buddhi*
  b) *aviśeṣa* = *asmitā-mātra* + five *tan-mātras* + *manas*
  c) *viśeṣa* = the empirical world being a compound of the gross elements (*mahā-bhūtas*) and the sense-organs (*indriyas*)

References to the ontological conceptions in the *Yoga-Sūtra* are few, but the little information given allows the following reconstruction: On the one side there are numberless transcendent and eternal Selves (*puruṣas*), on the other is the transcendent core of nature (*prakṛti-pradhāna*), the matrix out of which the whole manifested cosmos is created. Both ultimate principles are forever distinct and do not coincide, as the Upaniṣadic seers and particularly Śaṅkara announced. The first-born of the cosmic evolution (*sarga*) is the 'great' (*mahān*, *mahat*) or, if viewed subjectively, *buddhi*. Out of this develops *asmitā-mātra* (in Sāṃkhya *ahaṃkāra* or 'I-maker'), the principle of individualisation, and the five categories of fine-matter (*tan-mātra*) as well as the mind (*manas*). These, in turn, give rise to the five gross elements (*mahā-bhūtas*), and the two sets of five senses each. This ontological scheme may seem strange and confused to the Western mind, especially with regard to the mixing of psychological with cosmological elements, but it must be remembered that these metaphysical constructions are the result of meditative experiences and that they were formulated some twenty centuries ago by persons who had little interest in expounding sterile intellectual systems. They were merely to serve as sign-posts for yogins who set out to discover the Self, which is different from the universe. These scanty indications will have to suffice, but what is important for the present context is to know that there is a correlation between consciousness and world on account of which it is possible to experience the different levels (*bhūmis*) of reality by adjusting one's consciousness accordingly in meditation or rather in *samādhi*.

The lowest form of the enstasis is that which has a gross object (*sthūla-viṣaya*) as its support and in which occur certain awarenesses or ideas. It is called *vitarka-samādhi*.[109] The reason for the initial position of this *samādhi* is supplied by Vācaspasati Miśra:

> Just as an archer, when he is a beginner, pierces first only a gross and afterwards a subtle target, so the yogin, when a beginner, has direct experience merely of some gross object of concentration made up of the five [gross] elements, [such as] the Four-Armed [*i.e. Viṣṇu*], and afterwards a subtle [object].[110]

Vijñāna Bhikṣu explains that in this enstasis the yogin has direct perception (*sākṣātkāra*) of the gross form of the object of his concentration. He perceives it as it is, as it was and as it will be in future. He also beholds its near and remote features and even those unheard of and unthought of. Vijñāna Bhikṣu further states that the term 'gross'

[109] S. Dasgupta, *The Study of Patañjali* (Calcutta, University of Calcutta, 1920), p. 156, grossly misunderstood this enstasis holding that it is 'not as yet beyond the range of our ordinary consciousness'.
[110] TV I.17.

(*sthūla*) stands here for the elements (*bhūtas*) and the sense-organs (*indriyas*), and he warns us not to confuse this enstasis with auditions or visions in which heavenly beings appear to the yogin and communicate with him. In *samādhi*, he says, no conversation is possible.[111]

Having practised the first stage of *samādhi* for an adequate length of time, the yogin may suddenly find himself entering the next grade, the *nirvitarka-samādhi* which is bereft of the numerous awarenesses (*pratyayas*) characteristic of the first stage.[112] The gross layer of the object is now perceived as it really is, without accompanying ideas.

The progressive process of involution or turning inward in *samādhi* is, to a large measure, self-regulating. Thus when the natural tendency of the mind to turn outward (*pratyak*) has been counteracted by constant efforts in unifying the consciousness, so that it can easily be checked, the yogin is carried by a powerful current from one stage to the next, whereby the succession of the diverse grades must not necessarily be in conformity with the sequence of stages as outlined by Patañjali. The adept may, by the grace of the lord (*īśvara*) or through a special disposition, skip certain stages as was the case with Gautama, the Buddha, who had the experience of the last two *arūpa-jhānas* (Skt.—*dhyānas*) —the spheres of 'nothing-ness' and 'neither-perception-nor-non-perception'—before he was acquainted with the preceding six stages.[113]

By a regular development, the next stage the yogin should traverse after the *nirvitarka-samādhi* is the enstasis, having a subtle object as mainstay and being renewedly connected with awarenesses or presented-ideas, as J. H. Woods translated the term *pratyaya*. Patañjali designates this grade as *vicāra-samādhi*, that enstasis which covers all categories of the subtle realm of the cosmos, namely the five elements of fine-matter, the *manas*, *asmitā-mātra* and *buddhi* and even the primary energies (*guṇas*).

[111] *Vide Yoga-Sāra-Saṃgraha*, chapter I.

[112] Vijñāna Bhikṣu characterises the *vitarka* enstasis as connected with *vikalpas* or 'imaginations' consisting of a mixture of *śabda*, *artha* and *jñāna*.

[113] *Vide Yoga-Sāra-Saṃgraha* II: 'This [application by stages] is however only a general rule (*utsarga*), as remarked before, since by the grace of the lord (*īśvara-prasāda*) or by the grace of the true teacher (*sad-guru*), [the yogin] finds (*dṛśyati*) his own mind capable of abiding in the subtle stages at the very beginning [of his practice]. Then the previous gross stages need not to be practised by the one desirous of liberation, [for this would be] a waste of time.' Vyāsa (YBh. I.25) adds the following to this point: 'Though He [*i.e. īśvara*] is above [all feelings] of self-gratification (*ātma-anugraha*), yet [to Him] the gratification of living beings is a [sufficiently strong] motive.'

When in this enstasis the awarenesses or supramental 'thoughts' have come to a standstill, *nirvicāra-samādhi* sets in. Then the subtle object shines forth in its full light without being interfused by *pratyayas*. The highest modality of this enstasis is the state of *nirvicāra-vaiśāradya* in which the abyss of the soul (*adhy-ātman*) is utterly calm (*prasāda*).[114] Then transcendental knowledge (*prajñā*) is said to be 'truth-bearing' (*ṛtaṃbhara*),[115] now completely emptied of all 'imagining (*kalpanā*).[116] Here ends the inner journey of the yogin who set out to fathom the depth of the cosmos. He has traversed all the realms of nature and reached its ultimate ground. He must now proceed to withdraw completely from all objective realities, for the Self is not to be encountered within the compass of *prakṛti*. It is beyond the primary constituents, the world energies or *guṇas*, the most subtle aspects of the cosmos. The yogins who do not, at this stage, realise that World and Self are distinct realities and who accordingly do not conceive of anything higher, are called *prakṛtilayas* and *videhas*. Their liberation is but a pseudo-emancipation, for they are still within the reach of death (*kāla*) and the never ending round of rebirths.

There can be little doubt that both *ānanda-samādhi* and *asmitā-samādhi* are subdivisions of the *nirvicāra-vaiśāradya* enstasis, but very little can be said about them. The interpretations forwarded by the classical commentators and later interpreters are not satisfactory. Taking into account all the relevant information given in the *Yoga-Sūtra* itself, it can be inferred that both types of enstasis are phenomena of *nirvicāra-vaiśāradya*. Once the supraconscious fluctuations have been subdued, all that remains is intense joy (*ānanda*) and, on a higher level, the acute awareness of one's personal existence (*asmitā-saṃvid*). Vyāsa gives in his *Bhāṣya* (I.17) a systematic representation of the different stages of *saṃprajñāta-samādhi* which is not without interest here:

vitarka-samādhi	=	*vitarka* + *vicāra* + *ānanda* + *asmitā*
vicāra-samādhi	=	*vicāra* + *ānanda* + *asmitā*
ānanda-samādhi	=	*ānanda* + *asmitā*
asmitā-samādhi	=	*asmitā*

114 *Vide* YS I.47: 'When there is clearness in the *nirvicāra* [enstasis] [the yogin gains] serenity of the soul-abyss.' (*nirvicāra-vaiśāradye 'dhyātma-prasādaḥ*.)
115 *Vide* YS I.48: 'In this [serenity] the supramental cognition is truth-bearing.' (*ṛtaṃbharā tatra prajñā*.)
116 *Vide* TV III.3.

This table, reminding one of similar attempts in Buddhist literature, demonstrates very well the progressive unification of consciousness in *samādhi*. Of special interest is of course the *asmitā* enstasis, because it represents the last stage of the enstasis connected with *prajñā* or 'supra-knowledge'. If our interpretation of the *Yoga-Sūtra* is correct, then the basic feature of this enstasis is the constant discrimination (*viveka*) between the Self and the non-Self, that is, the subjective transcendent principle and the world. The knowledge born of this discriminative effort will carry the yogin beyond the ocean of this universe. In other words, he enters the *asaṃprajñāta-samādhi* in which all seeds (*bījas*) of conditioned existence are burnt out.[117] But before that can actualise itself, every attachment to wordly objects, even the discriminate vision (*viveka-khyāti*) itself, is to be abandoned.[118] This renunciation is called 'supreme abandonment' or *para-vairāgya*,[119] as distinct from the abandonment to be practised in the waking state.

While it is still possible to convey an impression of the essence of the *saṃprajñāta* enstasis, the *samādhi* without supra-knowledge defies description. Even those few who attain to this supreme level of consciousness are quite unable to put their experiences into words. But each of them confirms the utter 'other-worldliness' of this enstasis. Perhaps it is not without deeper significance that Patañjali calls it simply the 'other' (*anya*).[120] All we can infer from his work is that with the practice of this *samādhi*, the subconscious impressions (*saṃskāras*), the seeds of future births, are dissolved and with them all suffering (*duḥkha*). Vijñāna Bhikṣu comments: 'The enstasis (*yoga*) without supra-knowledge is [the same as] the inhibition of all whirlpools [of the mind]. Then residual subconscious impressions only remain in the mind (*citta*), otherwise [there would be] no possibility [of a return] to the waking state (*vyutthāna*).'[121]

This enstasis is said to last only seconds at first, gradually lengthening in time. Rama-krishna, the teacher of the world-famous Svamí Vive-

117 *Vide* YBh. I.18.

118 *Vide* YS III.50: 'Through renunciation even of this [discrimination between Self and world] [comes about], with the dwindling of the seeds [of conditioned existence], emancipation.' (*tad-vairāgyād-api doṣa-bīja-kṣaye kaivalyam.*)

119 *Vide* YS I.16: 'The supreme [form] of this [renunciation] is the thirstlessness for the primary energies [which arises] with the vision of the Self.' (*tat-paraṃ puruṣa-khyāter-guṇa-vaitṛṣṇyam.*)

120 *Vide* YS I.18.

121 *Yoga-Sāra-Saṃgraha*, chapter I.

kananda, however, remained in this exalted state for three days at first and later for six whole months at a stretch, which is nothing but an expression of his unusual genius, for three weeks are generally considered the most the physical body can endure without disintegrating.[122]

With the final phase of *asaṃprajñāta-samādhi*, which is termed *dharma-megha* or 'cloud of *dharma*', all fetters fall, the primary energies resolve into the transcendent core of nature, mind and body dissolve, and the long-sought liberation (*kaivalya*) is obtained. The Self (*puruṣa*) shines forth in full splendour. The yogin has safely crossed the threshold of relative existence. There is no new embodiment for him, no return to the wheel of conditioned existence.

The closed nature of this experience has bred some confusion in the minds of the native commentators misleading, in turn, the Western investigators. This becomes evident when one looks at the position they assigned to, and the definitions they gave of, the *dharma-megha* enstasis. In the *Yoga-Bhāṣya*, there is an obvious inconsistency with respect to the place of this *samādhi* within the sequence of stages,[123] a confusion shared by Vācaspati Miśra who shows little originality when it comes to the interpretation of statements regarding the spiritual path itself. His particular domain is philological analysis, which gives evidence of his being a scholar rather than a yogin. The following story, current in *paṇḍita* circles, would seem to support this view:

> In those days (as even today in part of Upper India), it would appear to have been customary to hold learned discussions on such occasions as marriages. Vācaspati, who listened to such a discussion on the occasion of his own marriage, was so struck by the vagaries of dialecticians that he resolved straightaway to devote himself to the task of setting forth authoritative expositions of all the darśanas. So great was his zeal, so mighty the task and such the patient and tireless devotion of his wife that the couple had grown old before Vācaspati could write finis to his labours. Then alone did Vācaspati realise the magnitude both of his neglect of his wife and of his wife's self-sacrifice; and as a tardy measure of reparation, he gave her name to the last and greatest of his works, so that she could live on

[122] *Vide* Swami Nikhilananda, *Ramakrishna: Prophet of New India*, abridged from *The Gospel of Sri Ramakrishna* (New York, 1942), p. 28.
[123] Compare YBh. I.2 with IV.29 etc.

perpetually in the *Bhāmatī*, though not in the bodies of children born of her. The story is so picturesque, so typical of the scholar's neglect and the true scholarly recompense, that it deserves to be true.[124]

Relying solely on the *Yoga-Sūtra*, avoiding all secondary explanations, we can say that the *dharma-megha-samādhi* has to be looked upon as a transitional stage transporting the yogin from relative to absolute existence. Even M. Eliade has failed to understand this:

> ... the 'cloud of *dharma*', a technical term that is difficult to translate, for *dharma* can have many meanings (order, virtue, justice, foundation, etc.), but that seems to refer to an abundance ('rain') of virtues that suddenly fill the yogin. Simultaneously, he feels that he is saturated and that the world is breaking up; he has a feeling of 'Enough!' in respect to all knowledge and all consciousness—and thus complete renunciation leads him to *asaṃprajñāta samādhi*, to undifferentiated enstasis. For the mystical yogins, it is at this stage that the revelation of God (Iśvara) takes place; ...[125]

Thus M. Eliade takes the *dharma-megha* enstasis to be a preliminary stage to *asaṃprajñāta-samādhi*. This is in full accordance with the arguments of Vyāsa to *sūtra* I.2. But it is contradictory to the evidence found in the *Yoga-Sūtra* itself and even in Vyāsa's commentary to some of the aphorisms of the fourth book, where he attributes this enstasis with the function of destroying the subconscious impressions and the subsequent bringing about of the liberation-in-life (*jīvan-mukti*); his exact words are:

> With the disappearance of the causes of suffering (*kleśas*), and the [fruits of past] deeds (*karmas*), the sage, even while living, becomes liberated. Why? Because misconception (*viparyaya*) is the [only] cause of the world. For surely, none has ever seen the birth of anyone free of misconceptions.[126]

Also, M. Eliade's interpretation of the term *dharma-megha*, which is again based entirely on the classical commentaries, is far from being

[124] S. S. Suryanarayana Sastri & C. Kunhan Raja, *The Bhāmatī of Vācaspati* (Adyar, 1933), p. x.
[125] M. Eliade, *Yoga: Immortality and Freedom*, p. 84.
[126] YBh. IV.30.

convincing. How can it be said, that in this state, the yogin is covered by a 'shower of virtues', when he has long transcended good and bad?[127] J. W. Hauer already objected against this construction, but gave no better alternative. Considering those aphorisms of Patañjali's work which deal with the final resolution (*pratisarga*) of manifested matter into the transcendent state of potentiality (*laya*), we may perhaps not be going too far, if we interpret *dharma* as *guṇa* or 'primary energy'. This is in need of a more exhaustive exposition.

According to Yoga-Sāṃkhya metaphysics, the whole universe in all its layers and dimensions is a conglomeration of innumerable *guṇas* or primary substances or energies. They are the underlying principles of all phenomena, of gross or subtle reality, material or mental. The word itself has three meanings, namely 'quality', 'strand of a rope' and 'secondary', all of which, as S. Dasgupta has shown, can be applied in the present context.[128] Hence it is not easy to translate the term by any one word. Different suggestions have been made, like 'subtle entities', 'qualities' or 'Weltstoffenergien', the latter stressing perfectly well the energetic aspect of these fundamental constituents of *prakṛti*.

There are three 'types' or 'modes' of these primary energies, technically called *sattva*, *rajas* and *tamas*—all again ambiguous terms, standing for the principles of clarity or light, activity and inertia respectively.[129] They are present in a state of equilibrium in the transcendent part of the cosmos, the unmanifest *prakṛti-pradhāna*. In fact, the eternal core of the universe is nothing apart from them. They are *prakṛti*. When this initial balance of power—the *guṇas* are forever in motion—is disturbed,[130] creation takes place by way of a progressive individualisation. Preponderance of the one or the other primary energy brings to life the diverse evolutes (*vikāras*), like *mahat* or *asmitā-mātra*, and so on. The function of the *puruṣas*, the transcendent Selves, during this process is to cast their 'light' into the first principle of nature. The

[127] *Vide* YS IV.7: 'The yogin's action is neither white nor black; [the action] of the others is of three kinds.' (*karma-aśukla-akṛṣṇaṃ yoginas-trividham-itareṣām.*)

[128] *Vide* Dasgupta. *A History of Indian Philosophy*, repr. (Cambridge, 1963), vol. I. pp. 243–4.

[129] *Vide Sāṃkhya-Kārikā* 12 and 13; YBh. I.2.

[130] The cause of this disruption is held to be the contact (which is not a real contact or *saṃyoga*) of the Selves with nature. In this connection, it should be borne in mind that *prakṛti* exists only for the enjoyment and emancipation of the innumerable *puruṣas*. The 'will' (*āśis*) to manifest for the sake of the Selves is inherent in nature.

reflection therein is enough to nourish the cosmic evolution. Thus the mere proximity of the Selves effects creation (*sarga*), while their withdrawal results in the dissolution (*pralaya*) of the manifested world. The problems inherent in this theory are obvious and, we may add, can only be solved by giving up the standpoint of absolute dualism and merging the *puruṣas* with the transcendent quarter of *prakṛti*. This would still allow a relative dualism, as we find it in Śaivism, which is of considerable importance for the Yogic *practice*.

To return to the point of departure, we can assume that *dharmamegha* refers to that condition in which the adept of Yoga has conquered all forms of conditioned existence, and nothing but the primary energies, the *guṇas*, in their non-objectified form are obstructing his final release. Like a rain-cloud, they cover his all-pervasive vision, but only for an instant of time, then the *guṇas* resolve back into the eternal bosom of *prakṛti*,[131] having served the purpose of restoring the original purity of the Self which now reigns in absolute freedom, or as Patañjali says, 'alone-ness' (*kaivalya*). This 'state' is beyond description. Any assertion must necessarily be in negative or paradoxical terms, like Yājñavalkya's 'not thus' (*neti*) or Vimalakīrti's 'thunderlike silence'. Patañjali rests content with declaring: 'Then the "seer" (*draṣṭṛ*) emerges in his true form.'[132] The 'seer' is, of course, no one else but the Self, the power behind the empirical consciousness or the *citi-śakti*. As in Advaita-Vedānta, this liberation is not real, for the Self is ever free, it is rather a becoming conscious of one's true identity. A comparison may assist the reader to grasp this point better. A man looks on to the surface of a pool trying to catch a glimpse of his reflection in the water. He gets more and more fascinated by this play, completely forgetting himself, with his attention fixed to the counterpart, distorted by numberless ripples. Suddenly he awakes from this hypnotic fixation recognising that he was duped by an illusion (*adhyāsa*). This is exactly the position assumed by Yoga, Sāṃkhya and also Vedānta.

Before this essay can be completed, one more point remains to be considered; this is the much-debated question of liberation-in-life

[131] *Vide* YS IV.34: 'Emancipation is the involution of the primary energies devoid of any purpose for the Self, or [it is] the power [behind] the mind standing in its true form.' (*puruṣa-artha-śūnyānāṃ guṇānāṃ pratiprasavaḥ kaivalyaṃ svarūpa-pratiṣṭhā vā citi-śaktir-iti.*)
[132] YS I.3: *tadā draṣṭuḥ svarūpe 'vasthānam.*

(*jīvan-mukti*). As we have seen, Vyāsa promoted the view that deliverance is possible even when still alive. But this standpoint is not sanctioned by the *Yoga-Sūtra*. Vyāsa, who was in any case not a follower of Pātañjalayoga, here introduced opinions alien to the radical dualism of this school of Yoga which makes no allowance for a liberation while yet embodied. As long as the Self has not cut all connections with *prakṛti*, it cannot be said to stand in its true form (*sva-rūpa*). What philosopher-yogins like Vaśiṣṭha or Śaṅkara taught as *jīvan-mukti* can, to the follower of classical Yoga, only mean close proximity to final emancipation. For him, as for Rāmānuja, release follows upon death, when the body has fallen off (*vi-deha*), and whenever a liberated person takes on a body again, either composed of gross or subtle matter, he is no longer residing in freedom, but is again subject to the laws governing the machinery of the universe. Even when residing in the highest and purest realms of nature, he remains subject to a thin veil of illusion (*māyā*), since *prakṛti* is *avidyā* or nescience. After having revealed the secret doctrines of Yoga, the composer of the *Kaivalya-Upaniṣad* finally declares:

> Through this, one gains the knowledge which destroys the ocean of the cosmic cycle (*saṃsāra*). Hence knowing this, one attains the fruit [of all efforts], the 'alone-ness'—one [surely] attains the fruit, the 'alone-ness' (*kaivalya*).[133]

[133] *Cf.* Plotinus' 'flight of the Alone to the Alone' (φυγὴ μόνου πρὸς μόνον), *Enneads* VI.9.11.

2 Some Notes on Ṛgvedic Interpretation

After a whole century of Vedic studies, Western interpretation and translations of the sacred scriptures of ancient India, and in particular of the *Ṛgveda*, their fountain source, still remain extremely far from satisfactory. Many prejudices, partly born of speculations about evolution, have militated against any deeper insight being directed into, or appreciation of, the philosophical thought underlying Vedic literature.

When the *Ṛgveda* fell into the hands of Western scholars, indology was still in its infancy. It is not surprising, therefore, to find that H. Th. Colebrooke, the first European scholar to write on the Vedas, completely failed to understand the importance and value of these earliest Indo-European documents of religious thought, holding that 'what they contain would hardly reward the labour of the reader, much less that of the translator'.[1] Several decades passed before Vedic studies were taken up seriously, the scholars now being convinced that Colebrooke's judgement was biassed and that there was a great deal to be gained from the Vedas, first as a philological key to Indo-European languages, and then as the foundation of later Indian thought. Invaluable initial work was done, to mention but a few names, by F. Bopp, F. Rosen and E. Burnouf who, through his lectures in Paris, inspired scholars like R. von Roth, Max Müller, M. A. Régnier and F. Nève. A host of others followed, among these J. Muir, H. H. Wilson, M. Bloomfield, H. W. Wallis, W. D. Whitney, A. Ludwig, E. W. Hopkins, P. Regnaud, A. Bergaigne, A. A. Macdonell, A. B. Keith, A. Hillebrandt, K. F. Geldner. Standing between the earliest school and the latest, we have L. Renou following more or less the traditional trend of interpretation, yet showing a deeper appreciation of basic Indian philosophical concepts. During the last two decades, however,

[1] H. Th. Colebrooke, 'On the Vedas, or Sacred Writings of the Hindus', in *Asiatic Researches*, VIII (1805), pp. 369–476.

there has been quite a perceptible shift towards a better grasp of and insight into what French scholars somewhat derogatorily used to term Vedic *fatras* or hotch potch, mainly thanks to the meticulous, deeply thought out work of J. Gonda and that of Jean Herbert who was bold enough to have turned to the Hindu sages themselves to probe their scriptures, thus breaking the tradition set by earlier scholars who thought they knew better than the Hindus, an attitude summed up, for instance, by Paul Regnaud in his declaration: 'Brahmanism is a product of ill-understood Vedism, that is to say, a Vedism haphazardly commented upon at a time when the original sense was lost.'[2] The expression *mal compris* strikes the keynote of Western presumptuousness. We do not deny that the essential meaning may at one time or another have been lost; Sāyaṇa's[3] commentaries for example bear witness to such a loss. On the other hand, it is extremely possible that the spiritual meaning of the Vedas has been kept secret from generation to generation by the true *brāhmaṇas*. We only know for sure that modern exegesis is neither profounder nor of a higher order than classical Indian exegesis.

Vedic Sanskrit or *ārṣa* was at first something like the Hittite hieroglyphs to such scholars as F. Hrozný and F. Sommer when the code had been deciphered. Hopes were raised after the discovery of Sāyaṇa's commentary to the *Ṛgveda*, and H. H. Wilson even thought that this work made no further material necessary, providing all essentials for a proper understanding of the *saṃhitā*, the 'collection' of hymns. Of a different opinion was R. von Roth, the founder of Vedic philology, who was not at all satisfied with the explanations of Sāyaṇa, given after all, some three thousand or more years later. Roth wanted to ascertain the meaning of the words of the *Ṛgveda* as intended by the Vedic *ṛṣis* themselves. However, to a great extent he neglected native traditions, discarding them as late productions only. Contemporary scholarship is perhaps a little wiser in having recourse to comparative sciences as well as, in certain instances, to the notions current in India. No doubt, tremendous progress has been made since Wilson first rendered the *Ṛgveda* into English (1850ff) and yet Roth's aim, to

[2] P. Regnaud, 'Le Rig Véda et les origines de la mythologie indo-européenne', *Musée Guimet. Annales*, I (1892), p. 58.

[3] Sāyaṇa, who lived in the 14th century, wrote commentaries on the *Ṛgveda*, *Aitareya-Brāhmaṇa*, *Aitareya-Āraṇyaka*, *Taittirīya-Saṃhitā*, and *Brāhmaṇa-Āraṇyaka* as well as a number of other works.

understand the Vedas in the original meaning, has so far found little attention.

For more than a century Western scholars have read in the Vedas exactly what their preconceptions dictated and have shown remarkable lack of intuitive insight. They thus left their successors a legacy rich in philological analysis and research into the intricacies of what one may call pre-historic data, but remarkably poor in interpretative elucidations, let alone in spiritual perception. Philological discussions, as necessary as they are, cannot exhaust the meaning of the Vedic hymns; more often than not they obscure it. After studying and analysing the words, we now have to take up the study of the meaning and value of the hymns, to pierce through to their inner content, the message contained in them, to appreciate their character of revelation (*veda*). We do not mean to abandon philological or historical research, but it is to be realised that all these efforts will, in the end, remain fruitless and frigid if the deep inner meaning of the spiritual songs of the ancient *ṛṣis* is not brought to life, if the thought behind the letter is not revived.

Unwilling as they averred themselves to read anything except their own or anthropology's latest doctrines, scholars lost complete sight of the incontrovertible fact that the teachings of the Vedas as scriptures and as having been so considered for thousands of years by countless generations of Indians, are spiritual above everything else—and if spiritual then also symbolical; that the perennial criterion expressed in the Christian Gospels holds good for any scriptures, the Vedas included: 'The letter killeth, the spirit giveth life.' Here two factors of importance intervene: in the case of the early Sanskritists, like H. Th. Colebrooke and H. H. Wilson, even H. Griswold, there was the Christian prejudice which blinded them to any truths that other religious beliefs might have to offer; in the case of the agnostics, or the purely materialistic school of thought, the sheer incapacity to read any religious message in the myths that confronted them is evident. It may here be argued that the scholars' aim was, above all, to explain the 'letter' and that this sufficed them. The trend of their exegesis, especially as summed up in Bergaigne, shows that this was not so by any means. They aimed at, and thought they had succeeded in, giving the whole meaning. If so, it may be counter-argued, an interpretation of a scripture must involve the 'spirit' as well as the 'letter'; the total ignorance of the former is quite a reflection on Western sagacity. The Vedas have been *killed* by those who gave out only dry bones, just as the Christian scriptures are killed by those who subscribe to their dead letter. Our essays on the *Ṛgveda* are a small attempt to restore some of that 'life' in as much as one may rescue it from the texts themselves, to revive that 'spirit' from a conception of life and cosmos so alien to our modern one, yet nevertheless so vital to the Indians themselves that the less sophisticated among them express the greatest amazement when they are told what Westerners have made of their Vedas.

Several gratuitous assumptions, or shall we say fallacies, which to this day have on the whole vitiated Western scholarship, are responsible for the lack of basic understanding evidenced in Vedic studies. First, that prehistoric man was *de facto* primitive; that therefore the earliest literature was, as a reflection of the primitive outlook, necessarily crude. (In this respect there is a constant confusion between primitive and prehistoric, which two terms are not necessarily the same; there are primitive people to this day among our highly sophisticated society, though superficial varnish may hide to a certain degree their primitive mentality.) Secondly, complete failure to realise that early humanity was of a psycho-mental constitution widely differing from our own, a factor of the utmost importance for the understanding of ancient Indian thought. Thirdly, absolute refusal to recognise the *ṛṣis* as the 'enlightened' poets or visionaries their descendants claim them to be, a refusal stemming both from the mistaken and prejudiced belief that 'primitive' means 'inferior' and that the so-called 'psychic' abilities are to be discarded as being expressions of a pre-logical mentality. We shall examine these points more closely.

I Trends nowadays are fortunately pointing towards a more intelligent appreciation of prehistoric man and of the mythology which is his spiritual legacy to us—mythology deemed 'futile' by Colebrooke, although worth studying because 'it influences the manners, it pervades the literature of nations which have admitted it'.[4] Indeed, it appears that the avant-garde of anthropologists has lately taken gigantic strides in trying to eradicate false notions. One evidence of a fundamental change in the idea of the so-called 'primitives' emerges from that excellent study *The Concept of the Primitive* edited by Ashley Montagu who contributed a substantial part;[5] and it may be hoped

[4] H. Th. Colebrooke, *Miscellaneous Essays* (London, 1837), vol. I, p. 4.
[5] A. Montagu (ed.), *The Concept of the Primitive* (New York, 1968).

that we are gradually getting away from that pernicious belief that prehistoric man was inferior to ourselves: 'In actual fact evolution does not occur by the budding-off, as it were, of "superior" forms from "inferior" forms, but by changes within a group.'[6] And: 'In point of fact most so-called primitive cultures are far from primitive and far from simple. In quite a number of respects such cultures are very much more complex than is any Western culture.'[7] Both the system of social relationships and the languages have been found to be far more intricate than our own. Similarly one doubts whether any of the later Indo-European languages shows such richness and complexity as Vedic Sanskrit. But an excellent example of prevailing attitudes is thus described by A. Montagu, and this could apply, with a change of one or two words such as 'Vedic concept' for art and painting, to attitudes evidenced by Western scholars when they tackled the Vedas:

> When an Australian aboriginal sketched the head of a man without a mouth, this was put down to his unsophistication, to his naïveté. That the aboriginal preferred to draw this way, that his art was highly stylised, and that when he wished to he could draw as well in the style of the 'civilised' world as any skilled artist of the western world somehow failed to be recognised . . . the learned world refused to accept the notion that . . . accomplished paintings could have been the work of prehistoric man . . . Both the refusal to admit and the reluctant admission constituted testimony to the fact that though this art might be the work of prehistoric man it was not primitive.[8]

A. Montagu, moreover, pertinently points out:

> One of the consequences of the belief that primitive man was so much less developed than ourselves is the failure to understand that prehistoric man of 15,000 years ago was, in some aspects of his life, capable of achievements which have scarcely been surpassed by men since.[9]

A similar extreme reluctance to admit the greatness of Vedic concep-

[6] op. cit., p. 157.
[7] op. cit., p. 159.
[8] op. cit., pp. 171–2.
[9] op. cit., p. 5.

tions runs throughout Western exegesis. But here, even more striking than failure of recognition, is the absolute incapacity to understand Vedic cosmogenesis as well as the meaning of the Vedic gods and the sacrificial rites.

II Those ethnical groups which to our day have not developed our ways of living and education show certain faculties of extra-sensory perception generally unexplained and derided by the modern sceptics.[10] Nevertheless such faculties exist as the data accumulated by the Society for Psychical Research demonstrate, but are generally more obvious in country people living in greater communion with nature (e.g. among the Scots and the Irish) than in urban people. The forceful development of intellect and the one-sided stressing it also securely close the door to 'psychic intrusions'. From the evidence gathered from those people whom we term 'primitives' and of whom many offshoots may still be found with their immemorial customs and peculiar ways of viewing life, it seems that prehistoric man lived in far closer contact with nature which to him was fully alive, that he 'read' into the heart of the latter and detected the vibrant pulse which he interpreted as lives at work behind the variegated forms. What with the help of imagination and the anthropomorphising propensities of human beings, one may well deduce how the various mythologies evolved. But we must remember that a myth is not a pure invention, but a fact or truth of mainly spiritual or psychological import, around which a story is built and keeps being embroidered upon as the centuries pass by. This factor is of utmost importance in the understanding of the Vedic invocations to the gods. For what the actual purport of the invocations which form the bulk of the Vedas might be, what the meaning of the gods themselves, their plurality and underlying oneness, what the cosmic significance of the Vedic sacrifice and conceptions of divine order could be, depend upon such an understanding but have been completely missed by scholars and in far too many cases merely reduced to meteorology or the rudiments of astronomy.

Here again the work of such giants of psychology as C. G. Jung, or of such excellent scholars as M. Eliade, is slowly turning scholarly thought towards a more realistic or less prejudiced approach to the problem of

[10] To mention but a few of these ethnical groups: Zulus, Pygmies, Igluuk Eskimos and Australian aborigines.

archaic mentality and a deepening appreciation which may eventually lead to a real grasp of ancient conceptions and their vital expression, the myth. 'Myth', says C. G. Jung in his autobiography, 'is the natural and indispensable intermediate stage between unconscious [*sic*] and conscious cognition'.[11] It cannot be argued that we have passed beyond the stage of myth, the subconscious is as active within us as with our ancestors. Through our very constitution we cannot escape formulating myths, but today our myths 'have become silent' as to the great questions, for example, of God, of evil, of human significance. Science is giving us a 'merely exterior world', to use Jung's expression, but man is both subjective or interior and objective or exterior. For his own mental sanity he needs fulness, the coincidence of the opposites which make up his nature. The purpose of myth is to explain 'the meaning of human existence in the cosmos, a view which springs from our psychic wholeness, from the cooperation between conscious and unconscious [*sic*]. Meaninglessness inhibits fulness of life and is therefore equivalent to illness'.[12] The last phrase provides an excellent description of the modern demythologised world. Furthermore, as again Jung points out, 'it is not that "God" is a myth, but that myth is the revelation of a divine life in man'.[13] This is indeed the revelation of the Vedic seers and their contribution to the upliftment of humanity.

III This leads us directly to the last point: to poets, visionaries, mystics—and are not the *ṛṣis* all three combined?—concepts such as the infinite or the one life pervading all, vibrant through every form of nature,[14] the eternal sacrifice performed at the origin of the world and still continuing, the divine harmony (*ṛta*), the right or true (*satya*), which for us remain only at the level of ideas, are realities directly apprehended in the depths of one's innermost being or soul, the 'heart' (*hṛd*, German *Herz*), what for lack of a better word can only be called intuition. In the *Ṛgveda* several words for this immediate apprehension are employed, all emphasising seership, well brought out in this verse:

[11] C. G. Jung, *Memories, Dreams, Reflections*, transl. by. R. and C. Winston (London, 1967), p. 343.
[12] op. cit., p. 373.
[13] op. cit., p. 373.
[14] 'The fair-winged one, who is but one, inspired poets by their incantations shape in many ways.' (*Ṛgveda* X.114.5.)

> They polish their thoughts with heart, mind [and] understanding, for Indra, the ancient lord.[15]

There is no need for the mystic to search for a physical basis as a prototype to his vision, as some scholars, Max Müller in particular, were at such great pains to find; no need for any deductive logic, any reasoning from the particular and concrete to the universal and abstract. The mystics of all ages—and the *ṛṣis* are no exception—plunged into another dimension of which the mind has no real measure and afterwards only sought out a concrete symbol to express their 'experience'.

It would be apposite here to consider the meaning of the word *ṛṣi* and the many and most important implications to which it gives rise, implications once again missed almost completely. Attempts to trace the word to its origin have been innumerable, as is testified both in Indian classical exegesis and in later interpretation, Eastern and Western. A good summary is given by V. G. Rahurkar.[16]

The consensus of opinion points towards √ṛṣ ('to go'), either as *arṣa* ('to flow') or as *ṛṣa* ('to pierce'). According to Monier-Williams' Sanskrit dictionary it might also be related to *arc* or *ṛc* ('to praise'). What is of importance to us here is that whatever its origin, whether we trace it back to the root meaning of 'rushing towards' or of 'flowing with [knowledge]', the main idea implied from immemorial times has been that of 'seership'—the connection with √*dṛṣ* ('to see') being constantly emphasised—hence that of prophetic vision expressing itself in inspired diction, for that is the function of the *ṛṣi*: to express what he 'sees', and by the power of his expression to invoke the gods and possibly to make them manifest to men, thereby communing with them. We may surmise that cosmic processes such as are divined by the *ṛṣis* in a state of ecstasy or perhaps even enstasis,[17] which is the nearest European equivalent for *samādhi* (a word which does not occur in the *Ṛgveda*), are transposed by the seers from their supramental, to use Aurobindo's phrase, to their mental level by means of a peculiar type of speech potent in sound, so that ordinary men might mentally grasp the meaning and be emotionally affected by the combination of sounds producing *mantras*. In ecstasy, the *ṛṣi* gains supersensuous knowledge

[15] Ṛgv. I.61.2: *indraya hṛdā manasā manīṣā pratnāya patye dhiyo marśanta.*

[16] V. G. Rahurkar, *The Seers of the Ṛgveda* (Poona, 1964), pp. xii–xv.

[17] *Vide* introductory essay, p. 35.

(*prajñā*) as well as the right and the capacity to transmute it, so to speak, for others, so that they too, by some sort of repercussion at a lower level, might somewhat partake of his experience and insight. Hence because of this faculty which enabled the *ṛṣis* to 'see' (*paśyati*) or grasp the divine wisdom, the Vedas were considered to be eternal truth.

To summarise, the most important characteristics of the *ṛṣi* are seership and that power of invoking supersensuous entities, of evoking for others and expressing in suitable language what he has perceived in vision, so as to affect both the non-physical entities and the humans—vision-converted-into-a-hymn or word or eulogy, which is J. Gonda's translation of *dhī*.[18] This function and its full implications have only now been recognised, thanks mainly to the work of the just mentioned scholar. The 'hymn' as such is again and again a 'ship' (*nāva*)[19] or a 'chariot' (*ratha*), the latter a commonplace in the *Ṛgveda*. It is the concrete means of communication with the gods for the *ṛṣi*. So Yāska, in his *Nirukta*, says: 'A seer [is so called] on account of his vision (*darśana*). He saw the hymns [declares] Upamanyu.'[20] Such a power of communion implies the existence or reality of the gods, real enough to the *ṛṣis*, but quite outside the orbit of Western mentality and thus denied *a priori*, but without the understanding of which the Vedas remain more or less a closed book. We should in this connection quote Aurobindo's pertinent remark: 'The cosmic powers act and exist in the universe; man takes them upon himself, makes an image of them in his own consciousness and endows that image with the life and power that the Supreme Being has breathed into his own divine forms and world-energies.'[21] This in itself requires a study which in its complexity reveals that there is no such thing as 'the primitive' in the Vedas and thereby disrupts the common notion about the evolution of thought. Thought is revealed as complex in depth and breadth as among the Greeks, if one takes pains to probe the many allusions and the myths in which it is enshrined.

Thanks to his wisdom and purity of mind, the *ṛṣi* was reputedly able to see into spheres of reality different from the physical universe; he had gained this right by way of strenuous exertion (*tapas*); his work or

[18] J. Gonda, *The Vision of the Vedic Poets* (The Hague, 1963), pp. 137–8.
[19] For instance Ṛgv. I.46.7.
[20] II.11.
[21] Aurobindo, *On the Veda*, repr. (Pondicherry, 1964), p. 295.

utterances then embody the quality of his vision, truth. This was automatically accepted for the Hebrew prophets, but somehow true spiritual greatness was tacitly denied for the Vedic sages. True, the prophets thundered about the lack of moral rectitude among their people and rose to great heights of rhetoric, both of which, until the 1920's, were of greatest importance to the Western mind; the *ṛṣis*, by contrast, were more prone to sing of the beauties of nature in terms of incomprehensible gods which they invoked by means of an incomprehensible sacrifice for no apparent purpose except material wealth or martial supremacy. Or else, they spoke in what appears perfect enigmas. But this is where the understanding of the symbolism of the *Ṛgveda* and the key to its mythology are of the utmost importance and where we have, to this day, failed lamentably to fathom it, although their every thought and word sprang from a vision of cosmos rooted in order, harmony, and many a hint appears in the *Ṛgveda* itself to set us on the right track as to the hidden meaning:

> *Soma* is thought to have been drunk when they press the plant.
> [But] the *soma* whom the *brāhmaṇas* know, no one tastes. (X.85.3.)

> . . . No son of earth [ever] tastes of Thee. (X.85.4.)

> Many a one sees, but has not beheld the Word.
> Many a one hears, but hears It not . . . (X.71.4.)[22]

Has the latter verse ever brought to mind the Christian parallel?—

> They seeing see not; and hearing they hear not, neither do they understand. (Matthew XIII.13.)

'Those who know have wings', says the *Pañcaviṃśa-Brāhmaṇa* (XIV.1.13). It would be the height of absurdity to take this statement literally. Yet this is exactly what was tried again and again—to force a literal meaning where common sense ought to have warned the scholar there could be none. Since the *ṛṣis* are considered to be knowers of truth, wise men (*vidvaj-janāḥ*), then surely they must take us to realms which cannot be acceded to except by means of wings—and not merely mental, but spiritual wings. Here we must admit our disagreement with

[22] Hymn X.71 is one of the keys to Vedic sacred or symbolical language.

L. Renou who rather contemptuously rejects Śrī Aurobindo's Vedic symbolism thesis:

> We may reject the psychical explanation, which occasionally appears in native exegesis, and which Aurobindo tried to revive. According to this theory the Veda is a vast piece of symbolism representing the passions of the soul and its striving after higher spiritual planes: thus the Veda, we are told, ceases to be a barbarous and unintelligible hymnary. I fear that it also ceases to be a document of prehistory.[23]

Obviously the European knows better than the native who, in his homeland, is regarded as a *ṛṣi* himself. Here the question, apart from a possible confusion between prehistory and primitive, is: What do we really know of prehistoric mentality except what we can work out for ourselves in studying whatever archaic document may be extant. All ancient religions have used symbols to express spiritual truths for the simple reason that no such truths can be fully explained to the human mind save by means of concrete objects standing for the truths themselves, in other words, symbols or myths, the stories woven around these truths. It is our loss of the key or meaning, where these symbols are concerned, that accounts for our poor understanding of all archaic religions such as the Egyptian and the Vedic.

The human mind cannot operate except in terms of pictures or images; whatever concept one may formulate, it can be reduced basically to an image; an image is a symbol. The mind is the great εἰδωλο-ποιός, the maker of images. From this to idolatry there is but one step. But from prehistory to modern times, the human mind has worked in the same way. So we find Sir Arthur Eddington stating:

> If today you ask a physicist what he has finally made out the aether or the electron to be ... he will point ... to a number of symbols and a set of mathematical equations which they satisfy.[24]

He continues:

> That environment of space and time and matter, of light and colour and concrete things, which seems so vividly real to us is probed

[23] L. Renou, *Religions of Ancient India* (New York: Schocken Books, 1968), p.17.
[24] A. Eddington, *Science and the Unseen World* (London, 1929), p. 20.

> deeply by every device of physical science and at the bottom we reach symbols. Its substance has melted into a shadow. Nonetheless it remains a real world if there is a background to the symbols—an unknown quantity which the mathematical symbol *x* stands for. What do the symbols stand for? The mysterious reply is given that physics is indifferent to that; it has no means of probing beneath the symbolism.[25]

The archaic set of symbols was different, but nevertheless did exist. The *ṛṣis* set themselves the task of investigating the 'unknown quantity'. They found a means to probe beyond the seen and devised their own sets of symbols or myths to express what they discovered. They were not 'indifferent' to what lay beyond, but attached the utmost significance to it. This may be better understood in the light of what has already been said on the value of the myth. We wonder whether L. Renou has ever fathomed out the meaning of and the reason for the 'single chalice' made into a 'fourfold one' by the Ṛbhus,[26] the 'seven-rayed, triple-headed Agni',[27] the 'triple aspect' of the 'bull',[28] the 'six burthens' which the 'one, moving not away, supports',[29] the 'fire which Atharvan drew forth from the lotus flower',[30] the 'four divisions' of speech of which 'men speak only the fourth',[31] and many other such enigmas which are certainly not mere quibbles. Nevertheless, L. Renou himself admits (and this is, indeed, a step forward):

> The Ṛgveda is much more than an adjunct to ritual . . . The aim was to compose on a given theme . . . not introducing direct accounts of the lives of the gods so much as veiled allusions, occult correspondences between the sacred and the profane, such as still form the foundation of Indian speculative thought. A large part of Sanskrit literature is esoteric. These correspondences, and the magic power they emanate, are called brahman: this is the oldest sense of the term. *They are not intellectual conceptions but experiences* which have been

[25] op. cit., p. 24.
[26] Ṛgv. IV.36.4.
[27] Ṛgv. I.146.1.
[28] Ṛgv. III.56.3.
[29] Ṛgv. III.56.2.
[30] Ṛgv. VI.16.13.
[31] Ṛgv. I.164.45.

> lived through *at the culmination of a state of mystic exaltation* conceived as revelation. The soma is the catalyst of these latent forces.[32]

Here is a full recognition that the *Ṛgveda* cannot be read according to the letter, and in its deeper implications it does not differ very widely from Aurobindo's thesis which we understand in a broader sense than Renou seems to have done.

For these reasons we may well query whether the *ṛṣis* really prayed for a lot of wealth, booty, cattle, sons, rain, and not rather for spiritual riches (*ratna*), for the waters of heaven, not the physical sky, to flood the inner drought of the human heart when it feels desolate and dried up; for the sun of illumination to shine in the gloom of man's ignorance —'Let us meditate upon that celestial splendour, Savitṛ. May he inspire our thoughts', sings the celebrated *gāyatrī-mantra*,[33] which from immemorial time unto this day has remained the favourite prayer of the Hindu; for heroic souls or 'heroic power' (*vīravattama*) to face life's challenges and tribulations. Even here we are told again and again in perfectly clear language for what kind of wealth they prayed, as for instance in this invocation addressed to Indra: 'Bring us, lord of bay, steeds to make us joyful, celestial (*svarvān*) wealth, abundant, undecaying.'[34] Did the *ṛṣis* really fear the darkness, were they really afraid lest the sun might never rise again, as the Western commentators have made them out to be? Such absurd notions may, indeed, be peculiar to barbarians or genuine primitive peoples; but to imagine that men who were capable of rising to the heights of poetic vision, had not at the same time achieved a measure of control over themselves and their surroundings; that men for whom the cosmos was rooted in the divine harmony —'the flowing of the floods is law, truth is the sun's extended light'[35]— in which all actions were performed in ordered sequence according to the highest laws ever conceived by human mind,[36] men who were capable of giving out the basis of a philosophy which was to develop

[32] L. Renou, *Religions of Ancient India*, p. 10. The italics are our own.

[33] Ṛgv. III.62.10.

[34] Ṛgv. VI.22.3.—We may well wonder whether 'with spirit fain for booty' one may reach for 'life eternal' (Ṛgv. III.31.9). Griffith who has translated the verse thus does not seem to have noticed the flagrant contradiction.

[35] Ṛgv. I.105.12.

[36] 'By law the son of Aditi, law observer, hath spread abroad the world in threefold measure' (IV.42.4), 'Guardians of order' (V.63.1), 'Ye by eternal order govern all the world' (V.63.7).

and flourish and remain unsurpassed throughout the coming ages, to treat these men as crude almost barbarian bards and the products of their thought as the first prattling of infant humanity, can only be the result of absurd prejudices and would be incredible except that it falls in with the bias of the age, a bias only now being very slowly overcome.

We have not denied the *ṛṣis* beauty of poetry—at least in most cases. The mastery of a rich complex language is only too obvious. Not so the depth of insight. This has escaped us, and we have mostly toyed with the husk of the myths used to enshrine the seer's thoughts, leaving almost intact the kernel which alone contains their message. One of the most beautiful myths of all antiquity, whose origin can be traced back to the *Ṛgveda*, perhaps even beyond, the godly gift of the divine spark to man, the fire that burns low in every human being until such times as it may fully blaze forth into such a solar splendour as was visible in all the great sages—the Buddha and the Christ and the long line of the unforgettable Indian seers and *munis*, that purely spiritual gift we have reduced to the mere physical fire or lightning which time and again was but meant to be its symbol. Similarly, the interpretation of the many myths clustered around the legendary figure of Indra, his killing of Vṛtra, his releasing the cattle or recovering it from the Paṇis, although possibly rooted in historical data, has never soared beyond their face value or their absurd meteorological reduction.

However, to prevent any foregone conclusions, we do not believe that all the hymns—there are 1028 of them—carry a spiritual or symbolical meaning. Some clearly refer to worldly matters reflecting the cultural life of the Vedic people. Naturally, we also do not hold that all Vedic *ṛṣis* were of one attainment. Many of them were talented poets with deep insight, a few were outstanding seers in the true sense of the word. The *Ṛgveda* is the product of very different ages and people. Some hymns are extremely old, others again are later additions. Probably we shall never be able to determine the date of the one or the other. But all the available material can certainly be classified. We can decide what falls into the clearly mundane field, what in the philosophical and what requires a deeper study. For the *Ṛgveda* comprises the whole vast field of Aryan culture. Stanzas about gambling and highly symbolical accounts of creation, as well as jokes about priests being compared to croaking frogs, are contained therein. But even when such mundane activities as throwing the dice are mentioned, the ethical undertone is never missing, as an unbiased study of this ancient sacred scripture will disclose.

To us, it is significant that Indian tradition speaks of the origin of the Vedas as *apauruṣeya* or 'non-human'. This is not to mean that the formulation of the truths contained in the hymns are outside historical calculation. This statement refers to the truth itself. Vedic knowledge (*veda*) is beginningless, because it was conceived in the Absolute by the seers. Hence the Vedas are timeless revelation, the descent into the empirical universe by the transcendent. As long as this point is not accepted by the interpreters of Vedic thought, the spiritual legacy of the ancient Indian seers, perhaps the greatest religious contribution for mankind, will remain a hidden treasure. It is to these seers that can be traced the fundamental Indian conviction that any philosophical doctrine (*darśana*) must be based upon experience, transcendental knowledge. To quote J. Gonda: 'Man has, the Indians always believed, to acquire visionary knowledge of being, of the truth . . . of eternal values and not merely think with his brain'.[37] For 'pure reason . . . cannot reach "integral being" '.[38] This standpoint is of primary importance and, as apparent from the foregoing introductory notes, is rooted in the tradition bequeathed by the *ṛṣis*, namely speculations based upon transcendental insight (*prajñā*, *veda*). These seers sought out or looked 'towards an inspiration',[39] as J. Gonda brings out clearly,[40] before they declared anything. Indeed, the flash of intuition or vision, *dhī*, and the wisdom-thought, *manīṣā*, insisted upon again and again in the *Ṛgveda*, are keywords which cannot be overlooked. As J. Gonda observes:

> The emphasis seems therefore to lie on the possession of, or access to, special or supersensual knowledge, on the possibility of mental contact with the transcendent and on certain abilities in the 'sacred and sacral sphere' derived from these.[41]

J. Gonda, furthermore, connects *manīṣā*, the inspired thought, with 'yoga-power',[42] the science of the latter leading to great powers of concentration with all that this implies.

[37] J. Gonda, *The Vision of the Vedic Poets* (The Hague, 1963), p. 19.
[38] op. cit., p. 19.
[39] Ṛgv. III.38.1: *dīdhayā manīṣām*.
[40] op. cit., p. 52.
[41] op. cit., p. 50.
[42] op. cit., p. 54.

The *Ṛgveda* is thus not a mere collection of hymns of purely imaginative purport, crude in intellectual concepts, but the highly poetised expression of the spiritual vision of seers. Since we are not in a position to enter into such contemplative states so as to induce such realisations, it is not for us to question the reality of the *ṛṣis*' results as expressed in the hymns. We can but try to understand them, to give them credit for a sensible, but also spiritual, meaning, and in so doing compare their sayings with other sacred scriptures wherever the comparison can apply (and it does apply more than one may suspect), and where all else fails, to turn to the *ṛṣis* of modern India, for they are by no means an extinct species. Although they may express themselves somewhat differently, belonging to a different epoch as they do, the main burden of their teaching is doubtless in accordance with the ancient tradition of their forebears. The difference in question of details and descriptive epithets is of little importance here. It is the inner truth valid for all ages, in whatever language it may be clothed, we are looking for in any religious document. That the *Ṛgveda* lends itself to such a reading, the following essays on ancient Indian thought will endeavour to show.

3 *The Hymn of Creation. A Philosophical Interpretation*

I The Unmanifest was not then, or the Manifest;
spatial depths or heaven beyond were not.
What encompassed, where, who nurtured it?
What ocean, profound, unfathomable, pervaded?

II Death was not then or immortality.
Neither night's nor day's confine existed.
Undisturbed, self-moved, pulsated the One alone.
And beyond that, other than that, was naught.

III Darkness there was; at first hidden in darkness
this all was undifferentiated depth.
Enwrapped in voidness, that which flame-power
kindled to existence emerged.

IV Desire, primordial seed of mind, in the
beginning, arose in That.
Seers, searching in their heart's wisdom,
discovered the kinship of the created with the uncreate.

V Their vision's rays stretched afar.
There was indeed a below, there was indeed an above.
Seed-bearers there were, mighty powers there were;
energy below, will above.

VI Who knows the truth, who can here proclaim
whence this birth, whence this projection?
The gods appeared later in this world's creation.
Who then knows how it all came into being?

VII Whence this creation originated;
whether He caused it to be or not,
He who in the highest empyrean surveys it,
He alone knows, or else, even He knows not.

Of all the Ṛgvedic hymns, the celebrated *nāsadīya-sūkta* (X.129) has perhaps received the highest praise and the worst condemnation, according to the depth or lack of understanding of the commentators. Nevertheless, one may still wonder whether the full philosophical implications have been fathomed out and sufficiently appreciated by Western exegesis.

This ancient poem contains within its short compass not merely an outline of subsequent Indian metaphysics—it heralds the Advaita-Vedānta and the Sāṃkhya ontology—but also touches upon the core of mystical doctrines East and West, particularly the philosophy of Plotinus.[1] No later speculation, whether philosophical or religious, has ever gone completely beyond its range, or has ever solved the ultimate mystery of the Absolute which, in the poem, is left to silent contemplation. Considered in depth, it reveals the essence of all metaphysical thought.

About the seer-poet (*ṛṣi*) of this hymn nothing is known. To all intents and purposes he remains anonymous, as so many great figures of past ages who cared for the quality of their work rather than for themselves. That the hymn has been ascribed to Parameṣṭhin Prajāpati can mean only one thing, that it was revealed in the highest state of *samādhi* to a person endowed with the gift of formulating what he 'received' or 'saw'.

I *na-asad-āsīn-no sad-āsīt-tadānīṃ*
na-āsīd-rajo no vyomā paro yat,
kim-ā-avarīvaḥ kuha kasya śarmann-
ambhaḥ kim-āsīd gahanaṃ gabhīram.

The Unmanifest was not then, or the Manifest;
spatial depths or heaven beyond were not.
What encompassed, where, who nurtured it?
What ocean, profound, unfathomable, pervaded?

[1] Plotinus, very probably influenced by Indian thought, conceived the ultimate cause and source of all being as transcendent and unknowable. His only positive way of describing this indescribable *ens a se* was 'the eternal One' or 'the Good' (ἀγαθόν).

The first line, translated here 'the Unmanifest was not then, or the Manifest', strikes the keynote of the whole poem. At the outset a warning should be sounded. We cannot really apply the canons of logic, the laws of the concrete analytical mind, to the metaphysical thought of the *ṛṣis* as expressed here without risk of foundering in hopeless argumentation, or of drawing nonsensical conclusions. There is here no question of sense data or of empirical evidence such as is usually admitted as being the only reality. From the very first verse, the poet confronts us with that state of being, that ultimate of ultimates beyond all speculation, whence is the origination and whence will be the resolution of all things. He is straining to give us a glimpse of that primeval oneness beyond time, beyond space, beyond the sway of the opposites, that state of inexhaustible fulness (*pūrṇatā*) of which the finite human mind can catch but a faint glimmer. Yet the mind cannot be excluded if one is to explain anything by means of language. It must somehow grasp and express what transcendental awareness holds as pure knowledge. As Plotinus pointed out: 'The act and faculty of vision is not reason but something greater than, prior and superior to, reason.'[2] Hence the extreme difficulty in describing the content of the transcendental insight. Upon the testimony of the sages, the mind is, whilst struggling to understand and to express, all the time immersed in that infinite which eludes its every attempt at pinning it down. The only requirement to touch the Absolute is to transcend the mind, for the infinite dwells in the human 'heart' (*hṛd*).

> Its form does not stand in [the field of] vision; no one can perceive It with the eyes. Those who, through the heart [or] [transformed] mind, know It as thus standing in the heart, become immortal.[3]

The poem begins with the introduction of two important terms, *sat* and *asat*, which may be rendered as Being and non-Being. *Sat* is the immutable substratum of all that is. *Asat*, however, is here not simply non-Being in the sense of nothingness. This would be in direct opposition to the whole tenor of the poem. For there is implied that the opposite of Being is not sheer void (*śūnyatā*), annihilation, but

[2] *Enneads* VI.9.10.Throughout this essay we have used the translation by Elmer O'Brien, *The Essential Plotinus* (New York, 1964).
[3] *Śvetāśvatara-Up.* IV.20.

merely the opposite of Being *as we envisage it.* We know and experience limited existence, that which 'stands out' through limitation—even to use 'existence' as a synonym of Being is not quite correct: existence is but the outer aspect of Being.[4] We might observe in passing that *sat*, that which is, is the root of *satya* or 'truth'. But *asat* certainly does not mean the false, although it can, in certain contexts, express just that. In this particular metaphysical poem it doubtlessly refers to another form or kind of Being, unlimited, spaceless, timeless, of which man is unaware, hence to a state the finite mind finds itself incapable of conceiving and therefore tends to deny the possibility of its existence. H. W. Wallis rightly points out that *asat* must have held within itself the potentiality of *sat*,[5] otherwise it could not give rise to *sat*, nor can *sat* emerge out of nothing—although the latter may be considered *nothing* by the mind. H. W. Wallis goes further: 'It is not merely the non-existent, but may almost be translated the "not yet existing".'[6] In other words, it is that which is held potentially and thus has some kind of being—the *laya* state of later Indian speculation.

Sat may thus stand for manifested Being, *asat* for unmanifested. These were not, claims the seer-poet, and in this fundamental assertion he brings to our notice an utterly inexpressible, transcendent state beyond all possible realms of Being we can imagine, an ultimate, summed up significantly enough in the second stanza as the One pulsating by its own power, beyond space, time, limitation, out of all relation to the humanly known. To this there is a striking parallel in Eckehart who declares: 'Nothing hinders the soul's knowledge of God so much as time and space. Time and space are fragments, but God is one. Therefore, if the soul is to know God, it must know Him above time and space.'[7] A similar approach to the ultimate reality has been voiced by mystics throughout the ages. We might recall Nicolas of Cusa's confession: 'I have learnt that the place wherein Thou art found unveiled is girt round with coincidence of contradictories . . . 'tis

[4] The word *existence* as opposed to *essence* is here used as that state of conditioned or manifested being—manifestation implying relatedness and thus limitation, the latter implying incompleteness—which provides the data of our sensory perception. Being intrinsically is unconditioned. Empirically it is known only indirectly, through its conditioned aspect.

[5] H. W. Wallis, *Cosmology of the Ṛigveda* (London, 1887).

[6] op. cit., p. 62.

[7] Sermon 36. J. Quint's German edition.

beyond the coincidence of contradictories that Thou mayest be seen, and nowhere this side thereof.'[8]

The use of further negatives, sweeping and almost devastating as they may seem to some, only serves to enhance this affirmation of beyond-ness and other worldliness so strongly held in the poet's mind, and certainly has a far deeper meaning than most commentators, particularly so W. D. Whitney,[9] could find in their exegesis. The negative details which follow on in this poem do not 'dilute' the force of the 'absolute denial' of any and every manifestation, as is claimed by W. D. Whitney.[10] Here could be compared Plato's *Sophistes*, the main argument of which tries to establish the *existence* of *non-Being*! 'Let not, then, any one assert that we venture to speak of non-entity as existing in the sense of the contrary of entity; since long ago we gave up asserting the existence or rationality of any such contrary.'[11]

There was neither space nor heaven beyond space, continues the *ṛṣi*. *Rajas* can mean either 'space' or 'air' or even 'ether'; Monier-Williams' dictionary also gives heaven, here obviously referring to the sky overhead; whereas the word *vyoman*, translated by 'heaven', should be understood in the spiritual sense as that state of consciousness beyond the mental 'prison', which can only be described as pure bliss (*ānanda-mātra*). Even these imponderables were not, states the poet. There is obviously still that much doubt to the mind as to what could be when everything has been denied. Who or what held this all in germ?

'In whose shelter' (*kasya śarman*) is translated here as 'who nurtured it', because of the idea of protection in the word *śarman*; hence the nurturing mother aspect symbolised, in all ancient cosmogonies as also in the *Ṛgveda* and in this poem, by the 'waters' (*ambhas*). 'This all' (*sarvam idam*) or cosmic manifestation as contrasted to 'That' (*tat*), the Absolute, was then but 'unfathomable water', the ultimate state of matter or *mūla-prakṛti*, the matrix through which the cosmos is generated, a conception which is developed in the third stanza.

The word *tadānīm*, 'then' or 'at that time', calls for consideration. How can one speak in terms of 'that time' or 'time' at all when the

[8] *The Vision of God*, Chapter IX. Transl. by E. G. Salter (London, 1928), p. 44.
[9] W. D. Whitney, 'The Cosmogonic Hymn, Ṛgveda X.129', *Journal of the American Oriental Society*, May 1882.
[10] op. cit., p. cx.
[11] Transl. by R. W. Mackay, *The Sophistes of Plato* (London, 1868), §. 259.

state evoked is out of time, out of all relation to time? Time as the 'moving image of eternity', to use Plato's definition, is the objective, cosmic but for all that purely mental representation or mirror of the subjective, great 'breath'. There is here an indirect hint at that eternal rhythm of cosmic life expressed in the next verse as the 'great breath', that 'eternal recurrence' inwoven in the very rhythm of life, evidenced at every level of manifestation in time and space, but in a certain sense carried over and expressed as the alternance of 'states' of non-activity or unity and activity or multiplicity. 'At that time' refers to one of those alternate states in which all that had been conditioned, finite, manifested and therefore active in time and space had reverted back into the latency of the alternate state, fused as one into the heart of the ultimate in which all opposites are resolved. Thus the word *tadānīm* is not out of place.

This first stanza clearly anticipates the Indian philosophical idea of the 'days' and 'nights' of Brahma as well as the Sāṃkhya theory of involution (*pralaya*, *tirobhāva*) and evolution (*sarga*, *āvirbhāva*). The *ṛṣis* observed and then gave out what they 'had seen' (*apaśyanta*) in their visions (*dhī*) by means of poetry or *mantra*, often in cryptic statements which the philosophers in due time built into highly complex systems. Thus the Sāṃkhya teaches the dualism of spirit (*puruṣa*) and matter (*prakṛti*), that substance out of which the phenomenal world is moulded, emerging from latency into objective existence to serve the needs of the many spirits or Selves. Evolution here means 'increasing differentiation', so that 'what was an incoherent, indeterminate homogeneous whole evolves into a coherent determinate heterogeneous whole'[12] and thence back to dissolution or *pralaya*. Empedocles' theory of the alternance of 'love' and 'strife' could also be cited as it is based upon the same idea of cycles. With him the principle of strife divides or scatters all things apart to form a differentiated heterogeneous world, whilst that of love starts all things back to their primordial undifferentiated unity.

II *na mṛtyur-āsīd-amṛtaṃ na tarhi*
na rātryā ahna āsīt-praketaḥ,
ānīd-avātaṃ svadhayā tad-ekaṃ
tasmād-ha-anyan-na paraḥ kiṃ cana-āsa.

[12] B. Seal, *The Positive Sciences of the Ancient Hindus* (London, 1915), p. 8.

Death was not then, or immortality.
Neither night's nor day's confine existed.
Undisturbed, self-moved, pulsated the One alone.
And beyond that, other than that, was naught.

Here we are again confronted with the negation of the 'opposites'. In choosing 'death' and 'deathlessness', life spiritual and life physical, 'day' and 'night', the changing and the unchanging, motion and rest, *time*, the poet summarises what essentially constitutes manifested life to the human mind. Light and darkness, good and evil, birth and death, whether these be considered in their factual aspect of day to day experience or in their abstract or spiritual sense, make up the warp and woof of human horizons. But these are limits, stresses the poet, and the state posited lacks these demarcation lines. Also, these limits denote a mind of some sort to cognise them, but mind was not yet.

In the *Bhagavad-Gītā* there is a clear expression of the alternating cycle of rest and activity, creation and dissolution, in the life of the One:

From the unmanifested (*avyakta*) all the manifested (*vyakta*) [things] stream forth at the coming of day; at the coming of night they dissolve in just that called the unmanifested.[13]

Another celebrated creation hymn of the *Ṛgveda* sums up this same alternation in the life of the Lord of Being in these splendid words: 'Whose shadow is immortality, whose shadow is death.'[14]

The poet has now reduced everything to an ultimate One, and to show that in spite of all the negations he has so lavishly used, it is still 'life', though life transcendent, that he is positing, he now describes that life in a more positive way as the One that breathes breath-less, by its own power. Another paradoxical statement to tax human logic!

The mighty pulse of the cosmos, the great breath which means life in its deepest sense, for everything that lives breathes, however imperceptible or however differently from what we strictly mean by breathing[15]—and breath means contraction and expansion—this

[13] BhG VIII.18.

[14] Ṛgv. X.121.2.

[15] Even the minerals (which contract and expand and get *fatigued*), even the solar system, the distant stars have their own way of 'breathing'.

great breath is chosen as the one characteristic that never fails, even in that state of being which is beyond anything the human mind can conceive. The essence of all existence, all rhythms, all movements is contained in the great breath. Obviously, since it is soundless, windless or breath-less-breath, the poet is only trying to describe the very essence of what in manifestation is breath. Inherent power, inherent motion, breath. Breath is not an attribute, it is the essence of, it is Being. W. D. Whitney's remark that the *ṛṣi* of this hymn 'anthropomorphises his IT by making it breathe as if a living being'[16] shows a remarkable lack of understanding of the meaning of breath, rhythm, the core of life, as implied in the whole poem as well as in Indian philosophy in general, a characteristic peculiar to the whole of creation and not merely to creatures as such, a characteristic the poet takes to be rooted in the One.

The keynote has been struck. The seer-poet has done his utmost to express the inexpressible. To intuitive perception, he has succeeded in a masterly way. To the mere brain understanding, he has but heaped up negatives upon negatives, resulting in a meaningless denial. This is W. D. Whitney's conclusion. The poet, for the latter, 'deludes himself with the belief that by first denying absolutely everything, and then denying all but an indefinable something, he has bridged over the abyss between non-existence and existence'.[17] In the following it is hoped to show the fundamental meaning at the back of this negative approach which, moreover, ushers in the famous 'not this' (*neti*) of Upaniṣadic thought, where reality is stated as not anything that we can know about and thus does not stand comparison with anything. The ultimate reality or *brahman* cannot be 'seized' (*gṛhyate*), declares the *Bṛhadāraṇyaka-Upaniṣad* (IV.5.15). S. Dasgupta explains: 'He is *asat*, non-being, for the being which Brahman is, is not to be understood as such being as is known to us by experience; yet he is being, for he alone is supremely real, for the universe subsists by him.'[18] Here also Plotinus may be quoted to full advantage: 'This principle is certainly none of the things of which it is the source . . . But if you manage to grasp it by abstracting even being from it, you will be struck with wonder.'[19]

[16] W. D. Whitney, 'The Cosmogonic Hymn', p. cx.
[17] op. cit., p. cx.
[18] S. Dasgupta, *A History of Indian Philosophy*, repr. (Cambridge, 1963), vol. I., p. 45.
[19] *Enneads* III.8.10. O'Brien's translation.

III *tama āsīt-tamasā gūḷham-agre'*
praketaṃ salilaṃ sarvam ā idam,
tucchyena-ābhv-apihitaṃ yad-āsīt-
tapasas tan-mahinā-ajāyata-ekam.

Darkness there was; at first hidden in darkness
this all was undifferentiated depths.
Enwrapped in voidness, that which flame-power
kindled to existence, emerged.

The poet is now becoming more positive. In this particular context where the definite attempt is being made to go beyond any known data, there is in this idea of 'darkness hidden by darkness' another of such gropings after that which is 'beyond' (*para*)—that state of pure being which to the mind is darkness indeed, but to the spirit absolute light. As Eckehart confirms: 'Where reason and desire cease, there it is dark, but there God is shining.'[20] We should not interpret darkness to mean simply the opposite or the absence of light. In Greek cosmogony all things are also traced back to 'night', that abysmal darkness the mind cannot fathom. Darkness, in all ancient cosmogonies, comes before light—for light is also that which 'stands out' and hence signifies differentiation, manifestation, action.

Some commentators rightly take this darkness to be the matrix from which proceeds all manifestation. This is confirmed by the second half of the verse. 'This all', or objective manifestation, was then 'waters', the symbol of amorphous cosmic root-matter (*mūla-prakṛti*), the basis of all substance and all forms, the 'all-pervasive' of the *Śatapatha-Brāhmaṇa*, the nurturing mother aspect, the *χάος* of the Greeks, the 'face of the deep' upon which broods the Spirit of God as in Genesis. The idea is the same. The Greek *chaos* does not mean an indescribable medley of all things, but rather that matrix in which all things shall be moulded. It is translated here as 'depths' to avoid the literal connotation of 'water', which to the modern mind has lost its ancient significance.

V. S. Agrawala has an interesting commentary: 'The waters represent the principle of rest in which matter existed in a state of equilibrium and as an amorphous mass.'[21] Furthermore he states: 'The principle of *salilam* is the same as *āpaḥ* . . . It is primordial matter,

[20] Sermon 39.
[21] V. S. Agrawala, *Sparks from the Vedic Fire* (Varanasi, 1962), p. 64.

the unformed void . . . primordial *prakṛti* in which the Creator lays his germ.'[22] The 'waters of life' of Christian scriptures, apart from their specific meaning of the Word of God given out through the Christ, may have had just a touch of the ancient connotation of 'water', the mother aspect of creation through which life bubbles forth to fulness and without which life remains unmanifest. Śrī Aurobindo defines the word *salilam* as 'inconscient ocean' and says: 'The existence out of which all formations are made is an obscure, fluid and indeterminate movement.'[23] Hence the idea of surging billows at the root of the world.

Whether the undifferentiated substance or the surging billows of the previous sentence are equated with the void which enwraps the eternal pulse is here not exactly clear, but must be so, especially if one considers how 'matter', to the conception of early European scientists, a solid substratum underlying all phenomenal objects, through further observations is dwindling to particles of atoms formerly deemed indivisible though now found more and more divisible, to electrical charges, to even 'energy', soon possibly to vanish into the vortex of *citta*, mental stuff, as the Indians express it. V. S. Agrawala explains that *tucchya* is 'void or spatial cavity',[24] the cosmos in latency. Understanding this spatial cavity as the cosmic matrix which contains all in essence, then following his arguments, a further step may be taken: this matrix implies circumscription, a protecting 'shell', as he calls it, within which life will germinate; but circumscription also implies limitation. Out of the unlimited the matrix is formed—in what way will soon be evidenced—the circle is drawn and life is shaped into its multifarious forms. Similarly, out of the block of marble the statue is carved. Creation in this sense means self-limitation, not an adding to one's self, but a focussing of one's potentiality into a chosen, restricted field. But imposed self-limitation, however self-willed, does imply sacrifice, an idea so prominent throughout the *Ṛgveda*, and for that matter in all ancient cosmogonies, but so utterly misunderstood by modern exegesis. We might note in this connection that the same idea is present in St. John's Revelation—'the lamb slain from the foundation of the world' (XIII.8)—and that the ritual sacrifice of Vedic times may have stemmed from this conception rather than *vice versa*. Again the idea of contraction for later expansion appears here, although this

[22] op. cit., p. 9.
[23] Aurobindo, *Vedic Glossary* (Pondicherry, 1962), p. 97.
[24] V. S. Agrawala, *Sparks from the Vedic Fire*, p. 72.

expansion takes places so to speak in a different dimension. However, the significant point about the 'void', which brings to mind Eckehart's *niht* or 'nothing', concerns another aspect of the question. There is here a hint as to the great void—be the latter the veil of the essence of matter as apparent here or not—which stands guard upon the threshold of the ultimate reality to which man can attain. At the human level or microcosmically therefore, if that reality is to be apprehended in actuality and not merely in theory, all sense data and emotional, mental processes must be reduced to nothingness, to that emptiness wherein alone the Spirit can manifest. One must go through the void to find the divine ground of being; for only beyond the senses and thoughts, beyond the warring of opposites and multiplicities, beyond the void, which is but the threshold, the *ātman* abides in bliss.

'That which flame-power kindled to existence emerged' is a contracted rendering of the original so as to avoid the great awkwardness evident in all purely literal translations. The living principle in which is all power arouses from within itself the fire of creation. In other words, from the unknowable darkness 'that' (*tat*) which lay hidden by the void is aroused to creativity by *tapas*—a word never satisfactorily translated, for no single English word can be found with its profound implications. *Tapas* is far more than mere 'warmth' or 'heat' or 'austerity'. We have to turn to Indian commentators for any real understanding. A. Chandra Bose explains the word as having a positive significance, 'not self-mortification but self-awakening by activising the spiritual power within oneself'.[25] This is valid at the human level and also, by analogy, considered to be similar at the cosmic level. For *tapas* refers to that contemplative act which as a result of contraction or focussing to one point (*ekāgratā*) arouses to action the 'flame divine' or supreme creative energy, elsewhere in the *Ṛgveda* personified by Agni, till then in a state of pure latency; this macrocosmically and microcosmically. Śrī Aurobindo makes the following pertinent remark: 'The action of the Causal Idea does not fabricate, but brings out by *tapas*, by the pressure of consciousness on its own being, that which is concealed in it, latent in potentiality and in truth already existent in the beyond.'[26] Here is thus meant by *tapas* the release of the supreme creative energy by means of intensest contemplation at the highest possible level. Obviously, only a master of meditation could have

[25] A. Ch. Bose, *Hymns from the Vedas* (London, 1966), p. 8.
[26] Aurobindo, *On the Veda* (Pondicherry, 1964), p. 302.

conceived of such a process and chosen it as an analogy for describing the divine creative act. As such a knowledge is extremely rare in the West, it is not surprising that current interpretations are so very poor and betray such complete ignorance of fundamentally spiritual states upon which are based these cosmogonic explanations.

A somewhat analogical thought may have struck Plotinus when he considered the beginning of creation in terms of 'radiation': 'How are we to conceive this sort of generation and its relation to its immovable cause? We are to conceive it as a radiation that, though it proceeds from the One, leaves its selfsameness undisturbed.'[27] Here again we are at variance with W. D. Whitney who, in the whole of his criticism, shows a profound lack of understanding, even ignorance, of Indian metaphysics. First he is not sure whether *tapas* in this context means 'physical heat or devotional ardor, penance'. He opts for the latter sense. 'For no such physical element as heat plays any part in the Hindu cosmogonies, while penance, the practice of religious austerities is a constant factor in their theories.'[28] The complete lack of foundation of such a statement may be evidenced by any glance at Hindu cosmogonical references, as for example to Agni, the flame who underlies all creation, the dynamic energy released at the foundation of the world, who in the *Bṛhaddevatā* is called *agrajā tapas*, primordial heat, who sets the wheel of cosmos revolving, who in the *Kaṭha-Upaniṣad*, as the 'son of the two' poles from whom proceeds manifestation, is identified with the *tat*.[29] Hence the translation of *tapas* as 'flame-power', because the inherent power and the release thereof are of the nature of the flame and are the very essence of the highest contemplative act. The overtones of these Sanskrit words have no equivalent in the English language. In the *Maitrāyaṇīya-Upaniṣad* it is stated that the divine One 'generated heat. The heat is a person and a person is the universal fire (*agni*).'[30] The qualification of heat as a person may at first glance seem absurd, but it only means that the principle that animates all creation is a divine intelligence, Agni, the personified dynamic power of the Absolute.

Furthermore, Whitney, taking as he does *tapas* in the literal sense of austerity, a sense he cannot really understand, finds the performance of

[27] *Enneads* V.1.6. E. O'Brien's translation.
[28] W. D. Whitney, 'The Cosmogonic Hymn', p. cxi.
[29] *Kaṭha-Up*. IV.8: 'This verily is That.' (*etad vai tat.*)
[30] *Maitr.-Up*. II.6:

penance, used as an image by the early Indians to express the accomplishment of any creative act by the Absolute in its phenomenal form, as Prajāpati, a 'grossly anthropomorphic trait'. This is, of course, rooted in the basic misunderstanding of the word. Graphic metaphors can but be taken from human experience, and those of the present hymn are no worse than those found in the Bible.

The word *ābhu* gives some difficulty. F. Edgerton translates the verse thus: 'What generative principle was enveloped by emptiness—by the might of (its own) fervour, that One was born.'[31] To the term 'generative principle' he adds in a footnote: 'Literally "coming into being", *ābhu*; noun to the verb *abābhūva* "came into being" vss. 6 and 7.'[32] Thereby he is following Macdonell. The One for him 'begets all beings'.[33] In a footnote he adds: 'RV 10.129.5 seems to compare the act of creation to a sexual act.'[34] Knowing the Western, and especially American, bias for reducing everything to sex, we can but turn back to Plotinus, that perfect 'Advaitin' (though perhaps unknowing to himself)[35] to find an explanation of this idea far more in the spirit of the hymn: 'We have to remove from our minds any idea that this is a process like generation in time because here we are treating of eternal realities. We speak metaphorically, in terms of generation, to indicate the causal relations of things eternal and their systematic order.'[36]

Both the Western commentators diverge widely from the meaning ascribed to *ābhu* by Monier-Williams and such Indians as Sāyaṇa, Kunhan Raja and Agrawala, for whom *ābhu*, in the case of Monier-Williams, means 'empty' and in the case of the others 'the all encompassing' or the all pervading. Following the latter interpretation, the verse could be rendered thus: 'The all pervading was covered with the void, and by the power of *tapas* was that One born.' According to Agrawala both *tucchya* and *ābhu* are technical terms. '*Tucchya* is void and spatial cavity, i.e. the cosmos; *ābhu* is that which pervades on all sides . . . and denotes Brahman itself.'[37] He goes on: 'The particular portion of *ābhu* that was shadowed by *tucchya* generates within itself

[31] F. Edgerton, *The Beginnings of Indian Philosophy* (London, 1965), p. 73.
[32] op. cit., p. 73.
[33] op. cit., p. 25.
[34] op. cit., p. 25.
[35] *Cf.* O. Lacombe, 'Note sur Plotin et la pensée indienne', *École Pratique des Hautes Études*. Annuaire 1950–1 (Paris, 1950).
[36] *Enneads* V.1.6.
[37] V. S. Agrawala, *Sparks from the Vedic Fire*, p. 72.

the temperature of heat which brings into being the individual centres manifesting as the sun in the midst of each system. Sūrya is the manifest form of intense *tapas*.'[38] Sūrya, one may add, is the great ancient symbol of manifested Deity.

To sum up the meaning of this much debated verse. The *ṛṣi* conceived that through some analogical kind of concentration and contemplation as that known to human beings—an action which is first contraction to a focus—the divine life then expands into the activity of creation or manifestation by which the One pouring itself forth becomes the Many. Whilst through the veil of root-matter (*prakṛti-pradhāna*), whether unmanifest (*avyakta*) or manifest (*vyakta*) the great breath pulsates eternally.

IV *kāmas-tad-agre sam-avartata-adhi,*
manaso retaḥ prathamaṃ yad-āsīt,
sato bandhum-asati nir-avindan-
hṛdi pratīṣyā kavayo manīṣā.

Desire, primordial seed of mind,
in the beginning, arose in That.
Seers, searching in their heart's wisdom,
discovered the kinship of the created
with the uncreate.

The poet now becomes most specific. One should first notice the continual reference to the impersonal *tat*. The primordial One, the unknown darkness in which all is contained in latency, the infinite is simply 'That'—beyond attributes (*nirguṇa*), beyond mind and the senses. One should also compare the first line of this verse together with the preceding three stanzas with Böhme's curiously similar statements in his *The Signature of All Things*:

8. We understand that without nature there is an eternal stillness and rest, *viz.* the Nothing; and then we understand that an eternal will arises in the nothing, to introduce the nothing into something, that the will might find, feel and behold itself.

9. For in the nothing the will would not be manifest to itself,

[38] op. cit., p. 73.

> wherefore we know that the will seeks itself, and finds itself in itself, and its seeking is a desire, and its finding is the essence of the desire, wherein the will finds itself.[39]

Obviously, the Christian mystic, through his own contemplative absorption, arrived at the same kind of view as the Indian *ṛṣi*. Here again we have the 'nothing' to describe what is unfathomable to the mind.

Kāma, translated here by 'desire', calls for elucidation. J. Mascaró renders the word as 'love'.[40] This should not be considered, in the present context, as just desire for sensuous experience. The *ṛṣi* is treating of transcendental 'acts', and this should be constantly kept in mind. There can be no doubt, the word is here used in its highest connotation, just as J. Böhme also used the same word but without any reference to its mere earthly meaning. Love in its purest essence, as ἀγάπη, is desire and its own fulfilment: self-offering and self-fulfilment in the very act of self-offering. Nothing higher than this love can there be and possibly this is the kind of desire—the all-kindling flame which creates as an act of self-gift and in the act fulfils itself—that the poet has in mind. The Indian idea of eternal recurrence at the cosmic scale has been criticised as a reduction of the cosmos to a mere machine. The implications of the word *kāma* should dispel such erroneous impressions.

In the *Atharvaveda*, Agni is actually called Kāma who appears in IX.2 as the creative desire, the first born, whom neither gods nor mortals can rival. The myth is here quite transparent. Kāma is the essence of the divine creative flame and as such involves will, love, fire. Gods and humans are only partakers of this fire according to the measure that they also are divine. They can only create at their own limited level. Kāma is the concrete expression of *tapas*, the kindled flame resulting from the action of the latter, the divine will which by its *fiat* (let it be) caused manifestation; the ultimate product of *tapas*, *i.e.* the cosmos, is not illusory in the common sense, but it is also not completely real. Another typical Indian paradox! It is the Absolute or the One seen under a veil, hence the Indian idea of *māyā* which—apart from every meaning which has been ascribed to it by commentators

[39] Chapter II. Transl. by J. Ellistone, *The Signature of all Things and Other Writings* (London, 1912).

[40] J. Mascaró, *The Upanishads*, Penguin Books (Harmondsworth, 1965), pp. 9–10.

despairing of grasping its basic sense—signifies a 'measure' of reality, from $\sqrt{m\bar{a}}$ ('to measure, mark off, limit, apportion').[41] *Māyā* can be said to be 'illusion' only in the sense of veiling, or giving only a part of reality. Thus we may have a further inkling into the *Śatapatha-Brāhmaṇa's* paradoxical statement in connection with being and non-being:

> In the beginning this [world] existed as it were and did not exist as it were.[42]

The kernel of all later Advaita-Vedāntic thought is contained in these very early speculations.

One important point at this stage in the Ṛgvedic hymn under consideration emerges. Desire for sentient existence or that urge to manifest which is the one characteristic common to all aspects of life—however obscure or latent or unself-conscious in the atom or the plant, however fully or self-consciously developed, in man and the *devas*—is rooted in the very origin of life, in the primordial One. Thus the poet cuts the Gordian knot as to the eternal why of all this by ascribing this urge for life to the very essence of being: the need to be; it is inwoven in the rhythm of the one life and expresses itself in the recurrence of the 'days' of Brahma; the counterpart of this urge to activity being the urge to rest, the other facet of the eternal rhythm, the great breath of the One.

This eternal *why* has been the subject of speculation with man throughout the ages. Thousands of years after the *ṛṣi* of the present hymn, Plotinus also asked the same question: 'Why did the One not remain by Itself? Why did it emanate the multiplicity we find characterising being and that we strive to trace back to the One? . . . The eternally perfect is eternally productive.'[43] Once again the answer is that it is its own nature to create.

Desire (*kāma*) is stated to be the seed of mind. Desire, in its will aspect, is the propelling or dynamic force that moves to action; without it there is no activity. But before physical or material action can take place, there is mental action. Mind is the principle of differentiation,

[41] J. Gonda, *Four Studies in the Language of the Veda* ('S-Gravenhage, 1959). Chapter IV: 'The "original" sense and the etymology of Skt. māyā.'
[42] Śat.-Br. X.5.3.1.
[43] *Enneads* V.1.6.

the mover in action; it plans, directs, divides, puts order, shape, colour into a given field; it geometrises; hence manifestation is its handiwork. But it is the fire of desire or will that kindles it to action.

The Indian sages claim the mind is established in the heart. This is another way of putting what has just been explained. Macrocosmically, the universal mind comes into being only after *kāma*, the expression of the flame divine, has established a centre within the cosmic field, or the 'waters', or Aditi, the 'boundless' of Vedic cosmogony. From the unmanifest or heart of the One to the manifest or universal mind, that root of cosmos or differentiating power which produces multiplicity, there is but one step, brought about by *tapas*. Consciousness or universal mind cannot manifest before the flame, elsewhere Agni, here called simply *kāma*, wells up from within the depths of latent cosmic life, and by its impact upon the 'waters' kindles them to a mighty conflagration from which will emerge the starry galaxies. Combustion at the physical level is love at the spiritual level. The Christian scriptures maintain that love is the foundation of the world. But they are not alone in holding such a belief. The present stanza demonstrates that the *ṛṣis* also knew the fundamental meaning of love. Elsewhere in the *Ṛgveda*, Agni, the concrete form of *kāma*, is said to have entered the 'waters',[44] to have been discovered 'hidden in the waters' by the gods,[45] to have 'occupied, upright, the lap of the prone',[46] and to lie 'deep in the ocean . . . with waters compassed round about' whilst 'in continuous onward flow the floods their tribute bring to it'.[47] Agni 'waxes in the lap of the waters'.[48] Kāma indeed feeds upon the waters of life.

It is significant that the wise are represented as searching in their heart (*hṛd*) for the ultimate truth, not in their mind. As already explained, the mind can never apprehend truth as a whole, but the core of man alone touches the infinite.

A further difficult point is made. In their heart, the seers discovered the bond between that which is and that which is not, *sat* and *asat*, being and non-being, the defined and the undefined, translated here the 'created' and the 'uncreate' in order to avoid any misconception such

[44] Ṛgv. VII.49.4.
[45] Ṛgv. X.32.6.
[46] Ṛgv. II.35.9.
[47] Ṛgv. VIII.89.9.
[48] Ṛgv. X.8.1.

as usually arises in connection with these opposites to which we ascribe a definite concrete meaning.

Once again the logic of the mind seems to fail to grasp the link between the two. It is not explained *how*; there is merely the simple statement that this bond can be apprehended 'in the heart' (*hṛdi*), in other words, by soul awareness, not by means of empirical cogitation. Unless this be through intuitive perception—that flash of instant apprehension which occurs at rare intervals—we may *know*, in the deepest sense of the word, only when completely absorbed in that state of perfect at-oneness described by Plotinus[49] and implied here by the very expression 'searching in the heart'.

We are not surprised that W. D. Whitney can find no meaning in this verse. 'The verse seems to project, without any preparation, certain wise persons into the midst of the nonentity or its development . . . And wherever sat and asat, existence and non-existence, are brought together, it is a mere juggle of words, an affectation of profundity.'[50] Whitney notwithstanding, the mind can and does find some meaning here. It is not difficult to conceive of matter as ultimately energy, as explained in the commentary to the third stanza, and energy as ultimately mental 'stuff'. Hence the created is that which is compounded of particles of energy and like all compounded things will eventually be resolved into its constituent elements which themselves will be resolved into their original source. The created is thus rooted in the uncreate, in the 'waters' or essence of substance, the veil, or perhaps the breath of the One.

V *tiraścīno vitato raśmir-eṣām-*
adhaḥ svid-āsīd upari svid-āsīt,
retodhā āsan-mahimāna āsant-
svadhā avastāt-prayatiḥ parastāt.

Their vision's rays stretched afar.
There was indeed a below, there was indeed an above.
Seed-bearers there were, mighty powers there were.
Energy below, will above.

[49] 'The man who obtains the vision becomes, as it were, another being. He ceases to be himself, retains nothing of himself. Absorbed in the beyond he is one with it, like a centre coincident with another centre. While the centres coincide, they are one. They become two only when they separate.' *Enneads*. VI.9.10.
[50] W. D. Whitney, 'The Cosmogonic Hymn', p. cxi.

After his supreme effort to transcend the opposites, the *ṛṣi* now strives to visualise how differentiation arose. He could only express what he conceived in broad generalisations. We find general principles here, but nowhere is there a hint as to an anthropomorphic creator active in his creation. This is really a later simplification of the whole cosmogonic process intimated here.

This is perhaps the most difficult stanza of the whole hymn. Yet once again one does not at all agree with W. D. Whitney's sweeping condemnation that 'no one has ever succeeded in putting any sense into it'.[51]

The meaning of the word *raśmi*, considered by Macdonell as 'uncertain', cannot be taken literally. It seems rather to be a figure of speech. With their mind's eye or ray of inner vision, the sages probed the original undifferentiated substance to discover the broad principles as they emerged and first produced the division of the above and the below, the spiritual and the material, heaven and earth. Their yardstick was not a physical cord with which to measure the immeasurable, but the instrument of mental analysis which defines or delimits.

The poet refers to *retodhāḥ*, 'impregnators' or seed-bearers, and *mahimānaḥ*, 'powers', without any further particularisation. Macdonell and others describe these as 'male and female cosmogonic principles',[52] the positive and the negative powers, to whose action and interaction manifestation is due. The seed-bearers could be the gods who came into being as the embodiments of universal mind and who are the direct agents of creation in its details; seeds of the divine will which the many forms (*rūpas*) of the phenomenal world will carry within themselves; and the *mahimānaḥ* or divine energies could be their feminine counterpart or the *śakti* of Tantric philosophy. The phrase is very abstract and probably so with a purpose.

Agrawala has the following comment: 'The two principles essential for birth are the parental pair comprising Father and Mother. The Father is the retodhā and the Mother is the mahimānah.'[53] These two are constantly referred to in Ṛgvedic hymns as Heaven and Earth, the symbolic personification of the primeval parents.

C. Kunhan Raja in his commentary to this poem refers to 'spatial extension and life activity' as 'the two factors that arose in the infinite

[51] W. D. Whitney, 'The Cosmogonic Hymn', p. cxi.
[52] A. A. Macdonell, *A Vedic Reader for Students* (Oxford, 1960), p. 210.
[53] V. S. Agrawala, *Sparks from the Vedic Fire*, p. 75.

when there was the first activity of the mind'.[54] In other words, space and motion, the latter of which gives rise to time; space and time are inherent in the universal mind, but not in the ultimate reality. They are attributes of the mind.

The next line, translated 'energy below, will above', is quite intriguing and in the last analysis remains somewhat of a riddle. *Svadhā* means innate or inherent power or energy, and as it is coupled with the word 'below', the energy of matter, its own inherent nature must be referred to. But the word *prayati* is far more difficult as it is subject to various interpretations; its root is √ *yam* ('to extend, bring, produce'). Monier-Williams gives its meaning as 'offering, presenting, oblation, will' and Macdonell adds 'donation, intention'. C. Kunhan Raja translates it as 'activity'. For H. W. Wallis it usually has the sense of 'presentation of sacrifice' which is given in the dictionary as 'oblation'; this would explain the gods' action or act of creation at their own manifested level as an offering which would be in accordance with Ṛgvedic doctrines of the eternal cosmic sacrifice repeated indefinitely.

The word *prayati*, taken in the sense of 'intention' and with an eye to its root meaning of 'forth giving', may also imply the 'pattern' or 'intention' in the universal mind, the will aspect of the divine, concretised by the action of the gods or active agents or architects which these, in their quality of 'generators' or embodiments of the universal mind, bring down to the lower level or *avastāt*, below, to become the innate nature of each thing, the divine will made manifest. The whole problem of the interpretation of this stanza is still very moot.

VI *ko addhā veda ka iha pra-vocat-*
kuta ājātā kuta iyaṃ visṛṣṭiḥ,
arvāg-devā asya visarjanena-
athā ko veda yata ābabhūva.

Who knows the truth, who can here proclaim
whence this birth, whence this projection?
The gods appeared later in this world's creation.
Who then knows how it all came into being?

[54] C. Kunhan Raja, *Poet-philosophers of the Ṛgveda* (Madras, 1963), p. 228.

VII *iyaṃ visṛṣṭir-yata ābabhūva*
yadi vā dadhe yadi vā na,
yo asya-adhyakṣaḥ parame vyomant-
so aṅga veda yadi vā na veda.

Whence this creation originated;
whether He caused it to be or not,
He who in the highest empyrean surveys it,
He alone knows, or else, even He knows not.

The last two stanzas have often been taken as the proof of the final scepticism of the Vedic seers as to the ultimate truth. Do we really know how this whole cosmos came into being, asks the seer-poet, since there was no one to witness it? In the last analysis, we are ignorant of how the original processes of creation came about since no conditioned creature, no finite mind, could have taken cognisance of these and related the story. Even the gods themselves, the highest beings, who, however, are not forming part of the original *fiat* and come into being subsequently, cannot tell. We are only indulging in speculations which, at best, are approximations to truth. The whole reconstruction of the origination of the cosmos has, we believe, come to the *ṛṣi* in direct vision, in the deepest moments of *samādhi*; yet who is there to tell that he is right? The utter sincerity of the final question, 'who knows, who can here proclaim?', the humble, tacit admission that even the highest flights of illumination may fall short of reality, should be appreciated rather than smiled down at, as has all too often been the case. Thousands of years later, *we know no more*.

Throughout the poem it has been evident that the Indian idea of creation is quite different from the Christian conception. For the Indian speculation, creation is 'a letting forth' of that which was held in latency. This is fully brought out again in the use of the words *visṛṣṭi* and *visarjana*, both from $\sqrt{}$ *sṛj* ('to let go, emit, pour forth'). These two words summarise the whole doctrine of the projecting into more and more concrete expression of that which is ever latent in the inmost, a doctrine very close to that of Plotinus' *hypostasis*.

Two important points which seem to have been quite ignored by Western exegesis should here be noted. There is One in the highest heaven who surveys the whole world. Since he may or may not know the original process of manifestation, even he is not the Absolute, but deity manifested, the *īśvara* or 'lord' of later Vedānta. The use of the masculine pronoun *sa* or 'he' as against the primordial impersonal *tat* or 'That' is of the highest interest. It shows the dynamic pole of creation as himself a differentiation from the One, as one step down from unity towards multiplicity. In that ultimate unity the two poles, the active and the passive, lay as one, to be differentiated when the cosmic pendulum swung towards creation, separation, when the divine contemplation had reached such a peak that the *fire* of life was kindled, that the *fiat* of manifestation was sounded. Modern theistic religions have nothing beyond their active masculine creator which, to the Indian mind, is a finite god and thus only an aspect of that which is infinite or ineffable.

> Having pervaded this whole universe
> with one fragment [of Myself], I remain.[55]

This is the *Bhagavad-Gītā*'s summing up, a realisation inherent in the hymn of creation. Even that supreme overseer, the highest personification of manifested deity, muses the poet, may not know. The secret of it all may then be locked up in the Absolute beyond all godly grasp.

The second striking point on which no comment whatsoever has been made by Western exegesis, so far as we are aware, arises from the first. The poem ends on a similar note of transcendence as was struck at the beginning. Neither in the first stanza nor here is there any direct mention of the Absolute. That is left to intuitive perception. The final admission of human ignorance, and even of a possible ignorance on the part of the highest manifested deity, serves to elevate the idea of the Absolute, the One, the *tat*, to the loftiest heights the human mind can barely touch, to surround it with the utmost reverence and awe, beyond all speculation. The history of subsequent religion only shows a steady but complete degradation from the lofty estate to which the *ṛṣis* had elevated the Absolute. They had conceived and left It to the silence of deepest contemplation.

[55] BhG X.42.

4 *The Meaning of Suffering in Yoga*

In this essay an attempt is made to briefly examine one of the most important chapters of Patañjali's philosophy, the theory of the *kleśas* or causes of suffering, hitherto not given appropriate attention.

Although there are definite indications in both *Ṛgveda* and *Atharvaveda* that man in India was from the earliest times very conscious of the moment of suffering in the human life and interested in its metaphysical significance—this fact, the painful impermanence of conditioned existence,finds full recognition and elaborate discussion only at the time of the earliest Upaniṣads. Thus we can read in the old *Bṛhadāraṇyaka-Upaniṣad*: 'Everything different to this [transcendent Self, the Absolute,] is afflicted.'[1] The sage who is able to look behind the veil of empirical reality catches sight of the relativity inherent in the multiplicity of creation, which expresses itself most distinctly in the temporal limitation of all worldly objects. He fully realises the fatal cyclic movement—birth, life (illness, old age) and death—of all existing things,he clearly perceives the inner restlessness in the human heart, the confusion, fear of life, but also the urge for self-fulfilment, integration, perfection, and he wins the conviction that true fulness is only obtained by the estrangement from, and the surmounting of, the manifold and the powerful taking recourse to the transcendent (*para*), the *brahman*. Only complete identification with the Absolute promises emancipation from death (*mṛtyu*) and re-death (*punar-mṛtyu*). As the seer-philosopher of the *Śvetāśvatara-Upaniṣad* self-confidently declares: 'Only with the realisation of it [*i.e* of the Absolute] can one conquer death. No other path to escape is known.'[2] Furthermore he states: 'Those who thus know become immortal, but [all] others must

[1] Brh. Up. III.4.2: *ato'nyad-ārtaṃ*.
[2] Śvet. Up. III.8.

only endure suffering.'[3] The same seer speaks of traversing 'all formidable streams'[4] of the world ocean and thereby means the uncontrollable propelling forces of existence by which he feels himself overpowered.

The most frequently used Sanskrit term for suffering or sorrow in the philosophical sphere is *duḥkha* (Pāli *dukkha*), a word coined perhaps one thousand years B.C. in analogy to the Vedic *sukha*, meaning 'to have a good (*su*) axle-hole (*kha*), *i.e.* being comfortable, pleasant etc.'. The inner meaning of *duḥkha* is finely brought out in the *Nyāya-Sūtra* of Gotama: 'The characteristic of suffering is hindrance.'[5] There is a further interesting statement to be found in the *Nyāya-Sūtra-Bhāṣya* of Vātsāyana: 'When there is birth, there is pain; it is that which is felt as disagreeable, and is also known by such names as *bādhanā*, *pīḍā* and *tāpa*.'[6] Thus *duḥkha* is not merely physical pain, though in some contexts it may mean simply that, but it refers above all to the impermanance of the worldly objects and as such is of a deep metaphysical significance.

Though this 'painful hindrance'[7] is considered to be a basic fact in the cosmos, it would be totally wrong to suppose that such realisation led, on the part of the Indian sages, to an attitude hostile to life. It is true that the yogin to whom conditioned existence becomes transparent and who is able to discern the most subtle workings of, and relationships in, nature, does not display a fanatic thirst for life, but rather refrains from getting too much involved in its enticing-dangerous play. Although he endeavours to overcome *duḥkha*, he nevertheless does not consider it negatively. His point of view is in fact the same as that of Meister Eckehart, who expresses his conviction that the experience of suffering is not destructive but definitely positive in the following way: 'Note well, all pensive minds, the most fleet steed carrying you to perfection is suffering.'[8] In the *Mārkaṇḍeya-Purāṇa* the god-teacher Dattātreya declares: 'Knowledge comes about through suffering.'[9] This positive evaluation of sorrow contradicts the common Western notion about the 'Indian pessimism'. Indian philosophy does not end,

[3] Śvet. Up. III.10.
[4] Śvet. Up. II.8.
[5] *Nyāya-Sūtra* I.1.21: *bādhanā-lakṣaṇaṃ duḥkham.*
[6] *Nyāya-Sūtra-Bhāṣya* I.1.2: *tasmin-sati duḥkhaṃ tat-punaḥ prati-kūlavedanīyaṃ bādhanā pīḍā tāpa-iti.*
[7] This is J. W. Hauer's interpretation of the term *duḥkha.*
[8] *Von der Abgeschiedenheit.* Tract IX in F. Pfeiffer's edition of Eckehart's works.
[9] *Mārk.-Purāṇa* XXXIX.9.

as is so often maintained, in *Weltschmerz* or nihilistic despair. *Duḥkha* is 'painful hindrance' only to that person unable to attach any deeper significance to sorrow.

A thorough reflection upon the meaning of suffering in Indian thought is a prerequisite to any study of Yoga, for the painful impermanence of all things is nowhere experienced more intensively than in Yoga, where the adept, by constant efforts in changing his personality, lifts himself out of the valley of ordinary life with the aim of calmly and objectively examining the flux of empirical existence. As one who has, at least partially, overcome the whirlpool of human and cosmic affairs, the yogin's view penetrates the misleading façade of life and beholds the things as they really are: impermanent, painful, sorrowful. Patañjali has tried to put to these insights gained by the yogins a philosophical framework, and his thoughts on cause, meaning and termination of suffering, as sketchy as they are, build the fundament of classical Yoga and indeed any other form of Yoga.

Somewhat in the style of Buddhist writers, Patañjali expresses the all-presence of suffering in the cosmos in the following way: 'Because of the [moment of] suffering in the "vibrations" [of the psychomental life], in the affliction [of life], in the subconscious impressions and because of the opposite movements of the primary energies—everything is nothing but suffering to the one who discriminates' (*vivekin*).[10] With this, the author of the *Yoga-Sūtra* tries to convey that sorrow is a basic phenomenon of existence; it clings to all forms and modalities of the world and lies hidden in all things. But only the sage—Patañjali chooses the more adequate expression *vivekin*—is qualified to recognise this suffering hidden in the world. As the *Yoga-Bhāṣya* affirms, he is like an eyeball (*akṣi-pātra*) sensitive to the slightest touch of pain.[11] He sees through the sweet jugglery (*līlā*) of the cosmos; and all worldly pleasures, joys and delights become transparent to him, and he perceives behind them their painful impermanence, illness, old age, death —and finally new embodiment which sets this vicious cycle of suffering in motion anew. Sorrow is everywhere, even in joy, for behind it is always the anxiety of losing it and the fear of what may happen when the pleasure has faded. Not one of the many concealed aspects of suffering evades his sharpened perception. To him everything is rela-

[10] YS II.15: *pariṇāma-tāpa-saṃskāra-duḥkhair-guṇa-vṛtti-virodhāc-ca duḥkham-eva sarvaṃ vivekinaḥ.*
[11] *Vide* YBh. II.15.

tive, conditioned, 'painful hindrance'. Having established the universality of sorrow, he turns to inquire into the ways and means of overcoming this situation. As Īśvara Kṛṣṇa, the author of the *Sāṃkhya-Kārikā* states: 'Through the blows of the triple suffering [one comes to the] inquiry into the method of terminating it.'[12] The yogin's aim simply is to avoid all future sorrow.[13] There can be nothing more optimistic than this statement. The inquiry naturally commences with an analysis of the causes of suffering which Patañjali styles *kleśas*. The word *kleśa* (√ *kliś*, 'to torment, annoy, trouble') first appears in the *Śvetāśvatara-Upaniṣad* (I.11). It was known to the early Buddhists (as *kilesa*) and to the followers of Mahāvīra, the founder of Jainism. H. Jacobi identified it with the *doṣa* of the Nyāya tradition,[14] and he also stated that *kleśa* was from the beginning a *terminus technicus* of Yoga. As already indicated in the aphorism II.15 cited above, 'suffering' is woven into the very fabric of cosmic existence. Viewed objectively, it is conditioning, limitation, impermanence which, to the human mind, appear as pain, torment, affliction. Thus suffering is not purely mental, but based upon the processes and counter-processes which make up what is called the sorrowful ocean of the world. The more discriminating a person is, the more he perceives these fundamental antagonisms in the universe and the more he feels their impact upon himself, realising that he is like a small boat on the wild ocean. Patañjali now declares that it is this identification with the ups and downs of cosmic life and their influences on the individual which is the root-cause of all sorrow. In his own words: 'The correlation between the "seer" and the "seen" is the cause [of the future suffering which is] to be avoided.'[15] The 'seer' (*draṣṭṛ*) is of course the transcendent Self (*puruṣa*), and the 'seen' (*dṛśya*) represents the universe (*prakṛti*). 'The "seer", the sheer [power of] vision, although pure, looks upon the awarenesses [present in the mind].'[16] 'The "seen" has the character of brightness, action, inertia,

[12] *Sāṃkhya-Kārikā* 1: *duḥkha-traya-abhighātāj-jijñāsā tadabhighātake hetau. Cf. Sāṃkhya-Sūtra* of Kapila I.1: 'Now, the absolute termination of the triple suffering is the supreme aim of man.' (*atha trividha-duḥkha-atyanta-nivṛttir-atyanta-puruṣa-arthaḥ.*)

[13] *Vide* YS II.16: 'What is to be avoided, is future suffering.' (*heyaṃ duḥkham-anāgatam.*)

[14] *Vide* H. Jacobi, 'Über das ursprüngliche Yogasystem', *Sitzungsberichte der Preussischen Akademie der Wissenschaften*, XXVI (Berlin, 1929).

[15] YS II.17: *draṣṭṛ-dṛśyayoḥ saṃyogo heya-hetuḥ.*

[16] YS II.20: *draṣṭā dṛśi-mātraḥ śuddho'pi pratyaya-anupaśyaḥ.*

[and] consists of elements and sense-organs [and] has the purpose [of serving either the Self's] enjoyment [of the world] or liberation [therefrom].'[17] Brightness, action and inertia symbolise here the three primary energies or *guṇas*—*sattva*, *rajas* and *tamas*—and their respective appearances. The importance of this first fundamental discovery finds further elucidation in Patañjali's aphorism II.23: 'The reason of the apperception of the true nature of the power of the "mastered" (*sva*) and that of the "master" (*svāmin*) is [this] correlation.'[18] To this Vyāsa explains:

> The Self (*puruṣa*) as 'master' becomes correlated for the purpose of vision (*darśana*) with the 'seen', the 'mastered' [or 'owned']. The apperception of the 'seen' resulting from this correlation is enjoyment (*bhoga*). The apperception of the nature of the 'seer', however, is liberation (*apavarga*).[19]

Self and world, *puruṣa* and *prakṛti*, are eternally distinct principles. While the former is immovable, the latter is characterised by unbroken activity. False identification, *i.e.* the Self 'forgetting' its true identity and identifying itself with the mind (which is a product of insentient *prakṛti*), is the sole cause of all sorrow. The apperception (*upalabdhi*), another term for this mal-identification, results in world-enjoyment ('Weltessen', as J. W. Hauer renders the word *bhoga*) with all its fatal consequences. The apperception or realisation of the Self, on the other hand, secures liberation from the cyclic movement of birth, world-enjoyment, death and re-birth.

Thus at the base of all suffering is ignorance, namely ignorance of one's true identity. Patañjali expresses this fact as follows: 'The cause of this [correlation] is nescience.'[20] 'Is this [nescience] abandoned, the correlation is abandoned. This is the termination [of sorrow], the "alone-ness" (*kaivalya*) of [the faculty of] vision.'[21] The [faculty of] vision (*dṛśi*) is the Self, also called *dṛg-śakti*. Nescience (*avidyā*), the main cause of suffering, is said to be without beginning, since both

[17] YS II.18: *prakāśa-kriya-sthiti-śīlaṃ bhūta-indriya-ātmakaṃ bhoga-apavarga-arthaṃ dṛśyam.*

[18] YS II.23: *sva-svāmi-śaktyoḥ sva-rūpa-upalabdhi-hetuḥ saṃyogaḥ.*

[19] YBh. II.23.

[20] YS II.24: *tasya hetur-avidyā.*

[21] YS II.25: *tad-abhāvāt saṃyoga-abhāvo hānaṃ tad-dṛśeḥ kaivalyam.*

Self and nature are eternal entities.[22] Patañjali calls *avidyā* the 'field' (*kṣetra*) of all other causes of sorrow and bondage,[23] which are:

> I-am-ness (*asmitā*)
> attachment (*rāga*)
> aversion (*dveṣa*)
> thirst-for-life (*abhiniveśa*).[24]

Patañjali provides definitions of each one of these *kleśas*:

> Nescience is the [false] assertion of the permanent [being] in the impermanent, of the pure in the impure, of happiness in the sorrowful, of the Self in the non-Self.[25]
>
> I-am-ness is the seeming 'one-self-ness' [or identity] of the power of seeing [*i.e.* the Self] and that of vision [*i.e.* the mind].[26]
>
> Attachment is that which dwells upon pleasure.[27]
>
> Aversion is that which dwells upon sorrow.[28]
>
> The thirst-for-life flowing on by its own nature is rooted even in the wise.[29]

These *kleśas* are the root (*mūla*) of all 'work-deposit' (*karma-āśaya*) stored in the subconscious. They urge the individual to feel, think and act. These actions again leave, according to their nature, either positive or negative traces (*vāsanās*) in the subconscious which, in turn, have to

[22] Yoga and Sāṃkhya dualism cannot offer a more satisfactory solution to the problem of how the Selves came to be deluded by nature. Although a monistic philosophy, like Śaṅkara's Advaita-Vedānta, may interpret the relationship between Self and world in a more consistent way, the above problem remains also unanswered. It is one of the eternal riddles of existence which the human mind can never solve.

[23] *Vide* YS II.4: 'Nescience is the "field" of the other causes of suffering . . .' (*avidyā kṣetram-uttareṣām . . .*)

[24] *Vide* YS II.3: 'Nescience, I-am-ness, attachment, aversion [and] thirst-for-life are the five *kleśas*.' (*avidyā asmitā-rāga-dveṣa-abhiniveśaḥ pañca-kleśāḥ.*)

[25] YS II.5: *anitya-aśuci-duḥkha-anātmasu nitya-śuci-sukha-ātma-khyātir-avidyā.*

[26] YS II.6: *dṛg-darśana-śaktyor-ekātmatā-iva-asmitā.*

[27] YS II.7: *sukha-anuśayī rāgaḥ.*

[28] YS II.8: *duḥkha-anuśayī dveṣaḥ.*

[29] YS II.9: *sva-rasa-vāhī viduṣo'pi tathā rūḍho'bhiniveśaḥ.*

be lived out in the present life or in future births.[30] As long as the *kleśas* exist, birth, world-enjoyment (*bhoga*) and death and finally renewed birth are unavoidable.[31]

These causes of sorrow have two aspects; they can be either gross or subtle. Their gross appearance in form of *vṛttis* or mental activities is eliminated by meditation (*dhyāna*).[32] But their subtle form can only be removed by resolving the primary energies into the transcendent core of nature in the highest enstasis, the *dharma-megha-samādhi.*[33] In other words, the *kleśas* are overcome solely by the realisation of the Self, that is, by changing *avidyā* into pure knowledge or *vidyā*. When emancipation has not yet been attained, the *kleśas* may either be latent (*prasupta*, lit. 'asleep'), sublimated or attenuated (*tanu*, lit. 'thin'), temporarily suppressed (*vicchinna*, lit. 'cut off') or fully active (*udāra*).[34] It is the aim of *kriyāyoga* to attenuate these *kleśas* by means of *tapas*, *svādhyāya* and *īśvara-praṇidhāna* and thus to bring about *samādhi.*[35]

This progressive attenuation of the *kleśas*, the stimulants of sorrowful human existence, is the underlying process of all forms of Yoga. It is a consequent purification (κάθαρσις) introduced by a radical change of mind (μετάνοια). Having recognised that all sorrow is due to his own ignorance, the yogin makes every effort to remedy this nescience by careful discrimination (*viveka*) between Self and non-Self thus avoiding all negative, unwholesome thoughts, emotions, etc. He trains himself in the practice of the exact opposite of what the *kleśas* urge him to do. He replaces hatred by love, passion and attachment by serenity and

[30] *Vide* YS II.12: *kleśa-mūlaḥ karma-āśayo dṛṣṭa-adṛṣṭa-janma-vedanīyaḥ.*

[31] *Vide* YS II.13: *sati mūle tad-vipāko jāty-āyur-bhogāḥ.*

[32] *Vide* YS II.11: *dhyāna-heyās-tad-vṛttayaḥ.*

[33] *Vide* YS II.10: *te pratiprasava-heyāḥ sūkṣmāḥ.*

[34] *Vide* YS II.4: *avidyā-kṣetram-uttareṣāṃ prasupta-tanu-vicchinna-udārāṇām.*

[35] *Vide* YS II.1–2: *tapaḥ-svādhyāya-īśvarapraṇidhānāni kriyā-yogaḥ.—samādhi-bhāvanā-arthaḥ kleśa-tanūkaraṇa-arthaś-ca.*

As we have indicated in the introductory essay (*vide* p. 11), it is possible to re-organise the stages of Yoga in such a way that the importance of the two means of study (*svādhyāya*) and devotion to the lord (*īśvara-praṇidhāna*) is brought out better and that the techniques of *āsana*, *prāṇāyāma*, *pratyāhāra*, *dhyāna*, *dhāraṇā* and *samādhi* fall under the heading of *tapas*. If this sequence of stages is accepted, we must assume that Patañjali's original system is identical with this *kriyāyoga*. That *saṃtoṣa* and *śauca* are not mentioned in YS II.2 as parts of *kriyāyoga* may be accounted for by their secondary importance. They may well have been included in *tapas*. Otherwise, both terms may have been added at a later stage to the enumeration of YS II.32 so as to get the same number of entries for *yama* and *niyama*.

detachment, and so on. His continuous efforts cause powerful subconscious dispositions which are contrary to the *kleśas* and which serve the unification of consciousness, promoting his practice of meditation. The roots of the causes of suffering are finally eradicated by the practice of *asaṃprajñāta-samādhi*. Hence the following scheme results:

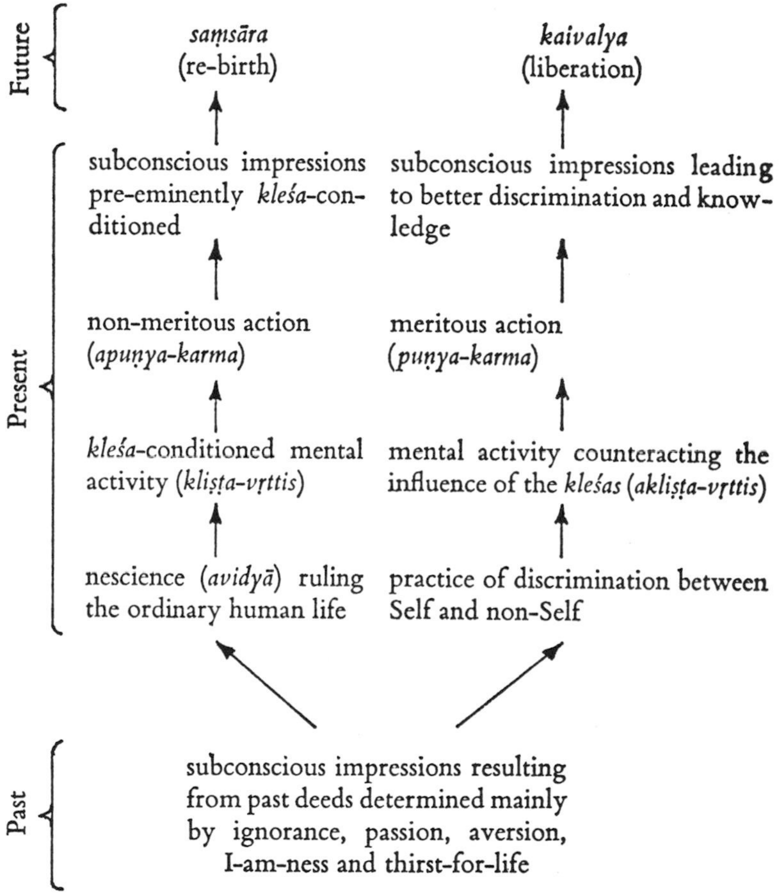

The above considerations throw new light on the gradual mastery (*krama-nirodha*) of the diverse contents of consciousness, revealing it as a threefold process:

1 The *kliṣṭa-vṛttis* or mind activities conditioned by the *kleśas* are substituted by
2 the *akliṣṭa-vṛttis* or mind activities counteracting the *kleśas*;
3 these are finally exterminated by *para-vairāgya* or supreme abandonment resulting in the *asaṃprajñāta-samādhi*.

The reason that also the *akliṣṭa-vṛttis* have to be abandoned lies in the fact that there is some element of sorrow even in them. Though they are conducive of emancipation, since they act counter to the *kleśas*, they are still within the radius of nescience or *avidyā* which has its root deep in the subconscious and which can only be dissolved by the continuous practice of the *asaṃprajñāta* enstasis, that *samādhi* in which all subconscious 'seeds' (*bījas*) are burnt out.

In this radical analysis of the subconscious, Yoga goes far beyond the Sāṃkhya which rests content with a mere empirical realisation of the distinction between *puruṣa* and *prakṛti*. The yogins have, at an early time, recognised the dominating role the subconscious plays in human life thus anticipating 20th-century psychoanalysis.

In conclusion we would like to remind the reader of the words of Geraldine Coster, psychotherapist:

> In the east *experimental* psychology has gone as far as if not much farther than with us . . . although yoga is perhaps an essentially eastern method, it nevertheless contains the clue needed by the west if the analytical method and theory is to reach its fullest scope as a regenerating and re-creating factor in modern life.[36]

[36] G. Coster, *Yoga and Western Psychology: A comparison*, 6th impr. (London, Oxford Univ. Press, 1957), pp. 9–11.

5 *Forerunners of Yoga: The* Keśin *Hymn (X.136)*

I The long-haired one endures fire, the long-haired one endures poison, the long-haired one endures both worlds. The long-haired one is said to gaze full on heaven, the long-haired one is said to be that light.

II The wind-girt sages have donned the yellow robe of dust: along the wind's course they glide when the gods have penetrated them.

III Exulting in our seerhood, upon the winds we have ascended. Of us, you mortals, only our bodies do you behold.

IV Through the middle region flies the sage shining down upon all forms; for his piety is he deemed the friend of every god.

V The wind's steed, the Lord of life's friend, is the god-intoxicated sage; within both oceans he dwells, the upper and the lower.

VI In the path of nymphs, angels, wild beasts wanders the long-haired one, the knower of heart's desire, a gentle friend, most exhilarating.

VII For him has the Lord of life churned and pounded the unbendable, when the long-haired one, in Rudra's company, drank from the poison cup.

This hymn is perhaps one of the most interesting of the Ṛgvedic collection from the point of view of Yoga. It gives us fleeting glimpses into certain aspects of Vedic religious life seldom mentioned elsewhere in the *Ṛgveda*, but more fully elaborated in the *Atharvaveda*. Few attempts have been made by Western scholars to elucidate its possible meanings and to place it in the main trends of Vedic culture. This may be owing to the fact that here are described certain feats too miraculous for the sceptic to consider or even understand, and certain beliefs which, at least in some quarters, would be deemed the field of the psychiatrist. Hence it was dismissed by M. Bloomfield, among others, as a panegyric of the sun rather than of human beings with extra-ordinary powers (*siddhis*). Only those investigators who, like M. Eliade, were concerned with its subject matter in a general way and were ready to consider its various claims and the authenticity of these, give us a sensible and well-studied insight into its data.

This hymn is indeed a eulogy on a type of ascetics who differed from the *ṛṣis* in marked respects and whose achievements are alluded to in the course of the description. To commence with, we are to consider the differences and the similarities between these ascetics and the *ṛṣis*. The latter—as one may gather from their invocations and praises—seem to have stressed sacrificial rites, and in addition to living a full social life, they probed the mysterious power of incantations and left as a legacy to their descendants hymns the full purport of which has not yet been fathomed by Western scholarship. The ascetics, on the other hand, seem to have developed more on the side of austerities and practices which align them to the later yogins. But both types had entrance into the spiritual order of the world, and their visions, in either case, are of a similar quality. One may thus agree with V. G. Rahurkar's broad differentiation of two main cultural strands in early Indian civilisation: the *ṛṣi* type, representative of Vedic Āryan thought which 'sponsored the Indra-cult, recited prayers and performed *homa*', and the *muni* or ascetic type which 'sponsored Rudra-Śiva cult', which V. G. Rahurkar considers indigenous and thus pre-Āryan, 'practised *yoga*, austerities and orgiastic rites . . . glorified life of renunciation, isolation and wandering mendicancy'.[1] The social organisation of Upaniṣadic India, whereby the life of the individual was neatly divided into *āśramas* or 'stages', may thus have owed its origin to the *ṛṣis*' social system, whilst the wandering ascetics of modern India may perhaps trace their ancestors right to the *munis*, *yatis* and *keśins* celebrated in the

[1] V. G. Rahurkar, *The Seers of the Ṛgveda* (Poona, 1964), p. xv.

Ṛgveda and *Atharvaveda* and of whom the longest description is here given.

Before studying the stanzas in detail, we should call attention to the very lively rhythm of the Sanskrit which is a characteristic peculiar to this poem, perhaps an attempt to catch by means of words something of the breath-taking flights, the exhilaration, the exulting mastery of the elements, of life itself, as apparent in these ascetics. Also, the economy of descriptive epithets should be noticed: each verse is pregnant with allusions which were probably quite sufficient for those who heard them in those days of recitation to evoke for them certain aspects of the ascetic life, indeed of life as a whole, steeped in a rich mythology as old as, or even older than, the *Ṛgveda*. Two myths, the churning of the ocean and the drinking of the poison, are specifically alluded to. But all these hints are lost upon us, their significance is buried in the dust of long ages, and we can only, by way of deductive reasoning and intuitive insight, try to recover part at least of their sense and content. Thus, after due consideration of its many implications and its lost significance, this hymn remains open to argument.

Tradition ascribes each of the stanzas to one of the *munis*, namely Jūti, Vātajūti, Viprajūti, Vṛṣāṇaka, Karikrata, Etaśa and Ṛṣyaśṛṅga, collectively called *vātaraśanas*, the wind-girt ones. So Sāyaṇa describes them as the sons of Vātaraśana. But only the third stanza is an actual quotation.

I *keśy-agniṃ keśī viṣaṃ keśī bibharti rodasī,*
keśī viśvaṃ svar dṛśe keśī idaṃ jyotir-ucyate.

The long-haired one [endures] fire, the long-haired one [endures] poison, the long-haired one endures both worlds. The long-haired one [is said] to gaze full on heaven, the long-haired one is said to be that light.

Here a very general description of the *keśin* or 'long-haired one' is given, and a short summary of his most outstanding accomplishments. From the second stanza, which identifies the long-haired one with the *munis*, we learn that the *keśins* are ascetics or holy men.

The word *keśin*, the epithet which describes the physical appearance of these ascetics, shows them as letting their hair grow and thus presumably differentiating themselves from other men, for it means primarily 'having long hair' and in this particular context refers to human beings. The word is also used to describe the flames of Agni, as they resemble long flowing hair[2] as in 'gold-haired Agni',[3] or for the streaming light of the sun, 'Sūrya with the golden hair'[4] or 'Savitṛ, golden-haired',[5] or for the radiations or fiery forces emanating from the *gandharvas*.[6] We must use our discrimination here as elsewhere, and we should not confuse the *keśins* of Ṛgv. X.136 with the triad of I.164.44. described by Sāyaṇa as Agni, Vāyu and Sūrya, or with any solar deity called *keśin*, as stated by A. C. Das,[7] or with the sun, even though this identification may be found in the *Nirukta* of Yāska.[8] In this work we can also find the following: '*keśin*: by hair, rays [are meant], *i.e.* endowed with these [rays] or on account of shining.'[9] M. Bloomfield, perhaps because of his inability to distinguish between the term 'hair' used literally when referring to men and 'hair' used metaphorically when depicting radiations whether physical or psychical, perhaps also through being influenced by Yāska's commentary, regards this hymn rather as a panegyric of Sūrya which 'is praised and compared to a muni';[10] if anything the opposite would be true, but the hymn has nothing to do with the sun as such.

Each stanza extols the *munis*, their ecstatic state, their essential goodness. We get a glimpse of certain types who, in later times, became peculiar to India, but whose counterpart are also met with in the dervishes of Islam, and of certain practices and their side-aspects which again, in due course, were to form part of the body of Yoga teachings. Nor can they be really regarded as only primitive shamans, as Oldenberg would have it. Their ecstatic state, as hinted at, contains an element of mental luminosity characteristic of the later Yogic experiences, and it is certainly worth studying each stanza in the light of the *Yoga-Sūtra* of Patañjali.

[2] *Vide* Ṛgv. I.164.44.
[3] Ṛgv. III.2.13.
[4] Ṛgv. X.37.9.
[5] Ṛgv. X.139.1.
[6] *Vide* Ṛgv. III.38.6.
[7] A. C. Das, *Ṛgvedic India* (Calcutta, 1921).
[8] *Vide Nirukta* XII.26.
[9] *Nirukta* XII.25.
[10] M. Bloomfield, 'Contributions to the interpretation of the Veda. II: The two dogs of Yama in a new role', *Journal of the American Oriental Society*, XV (1893), p. 167.

Yet there are some marked similarities between shamanism and the *munis*' experiences outlined here. M. Eliade, in his deeply studied work, defines the latter as a technique of ecstasy, the peculiar characteristic of which he summarises thus: '. . . special relations with "spirits", ecstatic capacities permitting of magical flight, ascent to the sky, descents to the underworld, mastery over fire, etc.'[11] Furthermore, 'The shaman is the great specialist in the human soul; he alone "sees" it, for he knows its "form" and its destiny.'[12] Each of these points should be kept in mind as we proceed with the examination of each stanza.

There is no intrinsic evidence in the present hymn that the *keśins* were a cultural group as well set apart as the *vrātyas* described in the fifteenth book of the *Atharvaveda*. It may rather be that the term *keśin* was applied to any person who answered to specific physical and psychological traits and practised certain austerities. However, R. N. Dandekar in his article 'Rudra in the Veda' distinguishes three religious cults or groups in Vedic times—the *vrātyas*, the *munis* and the *brahmacārins* as perhaps 'originally distinct from and independent of one another' and yet having striking similarities 'in point of ideology and practice.'[13] We may learn a great deal about these ancient ascetics by studying the *Atharvaveda* (particularly XV and XI.5), the latter being known as the *brahmacāri-sūkta*. The title *brahmacārin* is, according to Monier-Williams' dictionary, also given to a particular class of ascetics. The meaning of 'Vedic student' may have developed parallel with it or later, but it certainly does not apply to one who is described as 'quickening both worlds. The gods are joyful in him. He has established the earth and the sky',[14] as one after whom assemble 'the fathers, the god-folk, all the gods, the *gandharvas*',[15] as one who 'arose through *tapas* clothed with heat'.[16] This brings him rather in direct line with the *keśins* of *Ṛgveda* X.136 who also keep company with the gods and the *gandharvas*, and traces back the Indian veneration for the sage or ascetic to a very remote age and shows how in due time all sorts of miracles could be ascribed

[11] M. Eliade, *Shamanism: Archaic Techniques of Ecstasy* (New York, 1964), p. 6.
[12] op. cit., p. 8.
[13] R. N. Dandekar, 'Rudra in the Veda', *Journal of the University of Poona*, Humanities Section, I (1953), p. 101.
[14] *Ath. veda* XI.5.1.
[15] *Ath. veda* XI.5.2.
[16] *Ath. veda* XI.5.5.

to him, though certainly not to students. Nor could the *brahmacārin* any more than the *keśin* be identified with the sun except perhaps in a figurative sense as the bringer of light to other men, not in the absurd sense expressed by Bloomfield in his commentary: 'In our contributions . . . *Journ. Amer. Or. Soc.* XV.167ff., we have endeavoured to show that RV X.136 contains the glorification of the sun as a muni, a solitary ascetic: the present hymn [*Ath. veda* XV] may be understood best from a similar starting point. The sun who contributes elsewhere many of his qualities to the speculations regarding the primeval principle of the universe is here for the nonce imagined as a Brahmacārin, a Brahmanical disciple, engaged in the practice of his holy vows.'[17] In point of fact *brahmacārin* means the self-disciplined man, hence the ascetic. He is the 'one who wanders the path of *brahman*'.

The ascetic 'bears' or 'suffers'—with impunity, as one easily surmises—fire, water or poison, and the two worlds.[18] The meaning can certainly be taken literally, but there may also very well be a figurative sense which seems confirmed by the juxtaposition of the three nouns —*agni*, *viṣa* and *rodasī*,—and especially the last one. First as to the literal meaning. The mastery of fire is a feat quite common among certain types of people, like yogins, shamans and others. This is what M. Eliade writes on the subject: 'Magically increasing the heat of the body and "mastering" fire to the point of not feeling the heat of burning coals, are two marvels universally attested among medicine men, shamans and fakirs . . . One of the most typical yogico-tantric techniques consists . . . in producing inner heat ("mystical heat"). The continuity between the oldest known magical technique and tantric yoga is, in this particular, undeniable.'[19] He continues: '"Mastery of fire" and "inner heat" are always connected with reaching a particular ecstatic state or, on other cultural levels, with reaching an unconditioned state, a state of perfect spiritual freedom.'[20] One could also recall Patañjali's *sūtra* III.40: 'Through mastery of the [vital energy], *samāna*, [is produced] a flaring up [of the inner fire].'[21]

We may ask whether there is a profounder significance attached to

[17] Quoted by R. N. Dandekar, 'Rudra in the Veda', p. 100.

[18] The verb *bibharti* (from √‾*bhṛ*, 'to bear, endure') governs the three nouns *agni*, *viṣa* and *rodasī*.

[19] M. Eliade, *Yoga: Immortality and Freedom*, p. 106.

[20] op. cit., p. 332.

[21] YS III.40: *samāna jayāj-jvalanam*.

the fire mentioned in *Ṛgveda* X.136, a meaning akin to such age-old ideas as going through the fire or the fire of purification or particular ecstatic states. We may have in the expression *agniṃ bibharti* a hint as to the mastery of the *kuṇḍalinī* 'fire' which will be considered in connection with the fifth stanza. It is a fact that before he can be a master of life, as he is averred to be, the sage or ascetic must have gone through its trials—not merely physical but also psychological—and showed himself the master. If such were not one of the implied meanings, one might well ask why should he be said to bear the two worlds, as well as the poison. The *keśin* depicted here is not merely a fakir of Ṛgvedic India. The last two words, *viṣa* and *rodasī*, are a follow-on to the first, but certainly point to the fact that he stands above all things. We do not think that he purposely drinks poison for the sake of the feat, for that would not take him into 'heaven' (*svar*), nor would that entitle him to being called a light and the friend of every god as we shall learn soon. He can endure the poison of the world as well as being poisoned himself. For Yāska '*viṣa* is a synonym of water' deriving it from *vi-snā* meaning 'to purify'.[22] *Viṣa* means both 'water' and 'poison'. Philosophically, water was the symbol of matter, the great deep or substance aspect of manifestation. From such myths as that of Śiva drinking the poison of the world one might surmise the following: he who falls a prey to matter or materialistic ideals, becomes its slave; he has drunk too much from the waters of matter and cannot rise above them, he is poisoned. Not so the ascetic or the god who bears it or drinks it. We may now ask whether he takes upon himself the 'poison' of the world, the effects of the ill-deeds of mankind. This being the sense of the above myth, it may perhaps also be ascribed to the sage. The wording of the verse is so succinct that it is difficult to confirm or deny. But one may be entitled to consider the possibility, knowing that it is part of the true sage's *dharma* to receive and transmute the evil generated by human beings, a task summed up by a Ṣūfī teacher thus: 'We are the dustbins of humanity.' Further consideration will be given to this aspect in connection with the seventh stanza.

That the *keśin* can also bear the two worlds points to a detachment from life leading to its mastery, all of which raises him far above the rank of a mere fakir who may master fire, poison and such like, but may still be a slave to human passions, to the ego.

The word *rodasī* embraces 'heaven' and 'earth', *dyu* and *pṛthivī*.

[22] *Vide Nirukta* XII.26.

Rodasī, however, cannot mean just the two physical hemispheres, sky and earth, as generally understood by Western scholars. Śrī Aurobindo claims that *dyu* and *pṛthivī* refer, in the Vedas, to the mental or psychological and physical or material worlds, an interpretation which fits in with the tenor of this stanza. Sanskrit words have more often than not a broad connotation with specific meanings according to the context.[23] Discrimination is needed to see in which sense a particular word is used. Etymologically, *dyu* is derived from √*div* ('to shine, be bright, splendid'). This implies the light of the spiritual realms, the illuminated abode, the home of the 'shining ones' or *devas*. However, there seems to be a differentiation between the pure spiritual and the higher psycho-mental level of cognition. In this context, *dyu* would apply to the latter, and the former would be covered by the word *svar*. Similarly, *pṛthivī* has at its base *pṛth* ('to extend'), *prath* ('to spread, stretch'), *pṛthu* ('broad'), in other words 'extension', the philosophical term for matter, or the material world.

The *muni*, it is further stated, is not merely master of the two worlds, mind and matter, but he has penetrated into *svar*, the spiritual world or level of cognition. He can look beyond the body, the mind, even fully upon that divine light (*svar*) which one associates with heaven. He can gaze fully upon that splendour which would dazzle the ordinary mortal; he is even said to be that light (*jyotis*) in the sense of reflecting it on earth; he is that light, the verb 'to be' (*asti*) being understood. *Jyotis* is often used of the heavenly bodies. Monier-Williams gives these further meanings: the light of heaven, the celestial world, light as the divine principle of life or as the source of intelligence.

Svar, according to Aurobindo, 'means sun or luminous, being akin to *sūra* and *sūrya* the sun . . . *svar* is the plane of mental consciousness which directly receives the illumination of the sun *sūrya*. *Svar* is the name of a world of supreme heaven above the ordinary heaven and earth . . . Indra himself is *svarpati*—the master of *svar*, of the luminous world. It is the name of a world beyond the *rodasī*'.[24] *Svar* is given as derived etymologically as either from *su* or *sū* or 'according to some from a lost

[23] *go* or 'cow', for example, when in the plural means 'rays of light' as well as 'kine'; *ghṛta* may mean the essence of light or illumination as well as ghee thrown in the fire. While the last is not recognised by Western exegesis, the former is, through Sāyaṇa's commentaries.

[24] A. B. Purani, *Śrī Aurobindo's Vedic Glossary* (Pondicherry, 1962), p. 103.

root *svar=sur*, "to shine" cf. *sura'*.[25] One of the most beautiful incantations to Soma begs for that world of light:

> O Pavamāna, place me in that deathless,
> undecaying world wherein the light of heaven
> is set and everlasting lustre shines.[26]

This seems to be the 'heavenly' world to which the *keśin* has access, that state of ecstasy which the Vedic seers seem to have known and for which, as the hymn just quoted shows, they yearned. However, there is no evidence of a desire to escape from the physical shackles of life or, to use a later phraseology, from the wheel of births, a desire for absolute release or *mokṣa*. Rather the wish is constantly voiced that life be lived to its fullest length and in its fullest meaning. The *ṛṣis* were content with their visions of other realms of being and showed no urge to reach out beyond the world of manifestation, so marked a characteristic of their descendants. This same attitude is apparent in the *keśins* described in the hymn. Although they have tasted, or are constantly tasting, of that 'deathless undecaying world' (*amṛta-loka-akṣita*), they willingly accept the cup of poison from Rudra. In other words, they do not ask for liberation in the sense of Patañjali's *kaivalya*.

II *munayo vātaraśanāḥ piśaṅgā vasate malā,*
vātasya-anu dhrājiṃ yanti yad devāso avikṣata.

The wind-girt sages have donned the yellow [robe] of dust. Along the wind's course they glide when the gods have penetrated [them].

The *keśin* is here identified with the *muni*, without any commentary or explanation—everyone knows the *muni* is the long-haired one. *Muni* or holy man, from $\sqrt{\ }$*man* ('to think, reflect, perceive'), can be traced to the Indo-European *men* ('to think, ponder') and the Greek *μανία*. Later on the word acquired the significance of the 'silent one'.

The *munis* have only air for their girdles, are *vātaraśana* or 'wind-girt'. This may refer both to their utter poverty, willingly endorsed, and to their freedom from the barest necessities of life. However, the next few words might at first glance appear to contradict this if the meaning

[25] Monier-Williams' Sanskrit dictionary.
[26] Ṛgv. IX.113.7.

is pressed too hard. *Piśaṅgā vasate malā*, usually translated by 'clad in soiled yellow robes', the noun 'robe' being understood, is obviously pointing to the usual habit of these ascetics. *Piśaṅgā* is an adjective ('reddish, tawny, yellow') agreeing with *malā* ('dirt, dust impurity'). The verse thus literally reads: 'The *munis* are clothed in tawny dust', from which reading one would be entitled to infer that either their only robe is the dust of the earth or that they have donned the perishable vehicle of earth, the body, with all its impurities. Here we might recall the biblical statement as to the body made of dust, and to dust shall it return.[27] Nevertheless, in spite of this robe of flesh, the stature of the *muni* is such that he has achieved all freedom even that of the flesh, since he can ascend upon the wind as we next learn.

The wind, in its literal and figurative sense, has always played an important role in ancient thought. In Greek, πνεῦμα is either wind, breath of life and finally soul or spirit. So also is the case with the Latin *anima*. In Sanskrit there are two words for wind, *vāta* and *vāyu*. Vāta is definitely addressed as the god of wind in *Ṛgveda* X.168 and X.186, but only in these two hymns, otherwise Vāyu has preponderance. Aurobindo explains the specific function and significance of wind under the name of *vāyu*, and so further consideration will be given to it in our commentary to the fifth stanza where *vāyu* appears for the first time. In the present verse only *vāta* is referred to and may perhaps mean wind in the sense of *prāṇa*, breath-of-life, or of the Kabbalistic *Ṣēfer Yecīrah*, where it is said 'He maketh the wind his messengers',[28] or as in *Ṛgveda* VII.87.2 where the wind is qualified as the breath or soul or essence (*ātmā te vātaḥ*) of Varuṇa.

Upon the winds ascends the ascetic. He has the flexibility of the wind, he can rise upon its course—*vātasya-anu dhrājiṃ yanti*,—swift and light. We do not think that this should be understood literally, that he flies bodily through the air, although this, according to some authorities, is supposed to be specifically a Yogic power. Patañjali, in his *Yoga-Sūtra*, refers to this *siddhi* stating that levitation and 'non-contact with water etc.' follow upon the mastery of *udāna-prāṇa*, the life-energy located in the region of the throat and head.[29] It is more likely that here a flight out of the body is meant. We may again

[27] Genesis III.19.
[28] IX.10.
[29] *Vide* YS III.39: *udāna-jayāj-jala-paṅka-kaṇṭaka-adiṣv-asaṅga utkrāntiś-ca*. *Vide* also III.42.

turn to Patañjali and consider *sūtra* III.43, an aphorism which is more often than not misunderstood and which should be studied in conjunction with III.38. Translated literally it runs thus: 'The non-imaginary [psychomental] movement outside [the body] [is called] the "great disembodied" [or 'bodyless']; [when it manifests itself], then the covering of the inner light disappears.'[30] The 'non-imaginary' (*akalpita*) or actual outside-the-body movement of the mind is the subtle body (*sūkṣma-śarīra*) projected out of the physical shell. *Mahā* or 'great' does not necessarily mean physical greatness or spatial extension, but can well refer to the fact that in the subtle body there is no limitation regarding the speed and direction of the movement. *Vi-dehā* is indeed the body-less, *deha* usually being taken to mean the physical body. The 'dwindling of the coverings of the inner light' may refer to the fact that with the projection of the subtle body the sheaths of ignorance around the inner light are—to a certain degree—removed, for it confronts us with a level of reality unknown before. This kind of experience is far more in keeping with the tenor of the hymn as a whole. It is interesting to compare a verse of the Old Testament as translated by J. B. Taylor: 'And a wind raised me up and I heard behind me the voice of a great tumult.'[31] This phrase has also been rendered as: 'Then the spirit lifted me up and I heard behind me the voice of a great rushing.'[32] J. B. Taylor has the following commentary to this: 'Still in the context of his visionary experience Ezekiel was aware of being *lifted up* by the same divine impulse that had earlier raised him to his feet. (2:2) This was no psychic levitation, but a subjective experience of feeling airborne.'[33] Among mystics the actual physical levitation is a common occurrence of no importance and does not carry the body very far. The similarity between the Ezekiel description and *Ṛgveda* X.136.2 finds further ground in the next part of the verse where one can infer that the ascetic enters into those realms where the gods have penetrated; whether he is lifted up bodily or in the spirit, the result is

[30] YS III.43: *bahir-akalpitā vṛttir-mahāvidehā tataḥ prakāśa-āvaraṇa-kṣayaḥ. Vide* also YS III.38: 'The entering of the mind [*i.e.* the subtle body] into another body [is possible] by loosening the causes of bondage [between the physical and the subtle body] and by knowledge of the projection [of the subtle body].' (*bandha-kāraṇa-śaithilyāt pracāra-saṃvedanāc-ca cittasya para-śarīra-āveśaḥ.*)

[31] Ezekiel III.12. J. B. Taylor, *Ezekiel: An Introduction and Commentary* (London, 1969).

[32] Revised version, King James authorised and Septuagint versions.

[33] J. B. Taylor, *Ezekiel*, p. 66.

the same: he enters the godly realms just as the prophets did, the only difference being that the prophets acknowledged only the particular god of Israel and would have nothing to do with any others though occasionally others were mentioned. The last words of the verse under consideration, however, point to the fact that the gods have entered the ascetic, in other words, he is god-inspired. Hence, his capacity to enter the domains where alone the gods have dominion, as the fourth stanza will confirm. The whole point emphasises the freedom from earthly shackles and the kinship with the *devas*, ideas to be repeated throughout the succeeding verses.

III *un-maditā mauneyena vātān ā tasthimā vayam,*
śarīrā-id asmākaṃ yūyaṃ martāso abhi paśyatha.

Exulting in our seerhood, upon the winds we have ascended. Of us, you mortals, only our bodies do you behold.

As is frequent in Ṛgvedic hymns, we now notice a switch over from the third person to the first. The ascetics themselves are made to speak, to describe their peculiar state.

The emphasis once again is laid upon the ethereal side of their nature. The theme of the last verse is cleverly taken up and expanded, but this time the 'position or office of a *muni*' (*mauneya*), the exultation of his seership, are placed first and shown to be the one cause or the result of this ascension or standing upon the wind. Thus exalted the sage finds himself as light as air, as swift as the wind, as exhilarated as when a man is freed from heavy shackles.

We have ascended the wind, sing the *munis*, and only our bodies can you mortals behold. These words are quite significant, for they point plainly to the kind of ascension that is here meant. In the previous stanza only a hint was given, the meaning remained equivocal. It is now clear that the *muni* is able to leave the physical body at will, and ascend in the *psyche* to different planes or levels of reality. The physical body is left behind as a shell, visible to mortals, but the living entity is most active 'elsewhere'. The whole idea could be paraphrased thus: upon the wings of the inner breath we have ascended to realms which mortal eye cannot behold.

We have purposely refrained from describing these experiences or activities as 'in the spirit' but rather as 'in the psyche', holding that a clear distinction should be made between the Self, the spirit, and the psychomental apparatus (*citta*), the psyche. From the tenor of the following stanzas it is apparent that the experiences hinted at do not pertain to the highest stages of spiritual realisation; for there, as we learn from all mystical teachings, East and West, as well as from the *Yoga-Sūtra*, man transcends all manifested realms of nature (*prakṛti*), and he reaches out beyond all forms whether they be of angels or gods and achieves perfect union with the absolute reality, the unmanifest Self. The *munis'* experiences cannot even be regarded as simple states of *samādhi*; they still belong to the lowest part of the created cosmos.

Out-of-the-body experiences, consciously induced, are peculiar to Yogic and particularly Tibetan tradition, but by no means confined to these. M. Eliade makes the following comments to the *keśin* hymn:

> Some have wished to see the prototype of the yogin in this long-haired *muni*. In reality, the figure is that of an ecstatic who only vaguely resembles the yogin, the chief similarity being his ability to fly through the air—but this *siddhi* is a magical power that is found everywhere.[34]

We cannot completely agree with these considerations. There are various classes of yogins, and some of these do seem to fall in the category described here, especially if we interpret the flight as out of the body and not as a physical levitation. Eliade goes on:

> The description of his 'ecstasy' is far more significant. The *muni* 'disappears in spirit'; abandoning his body, he divines the thoughts of others; he inhabits the 'two seas'. All of these are experiences transcending the sphere of the profane, are states of consciousness cosmic in structure, though they can be realised through other means than ecstasy. The term is forced on us whenever we wish to designate an experience and a state of consciousness that are cosmic in scale, even if 'ecstasy' in the strict sense of the word is not always involved.[35]

The keynote of exultation which runs like a *Leit-motiv* throughout the hymn may give rise to the question why so much joy. From intrinsic evidence one might ascribe this to the sense of utter freedom,

[34] M. Eliade, *Yoga: Immortality and Freedom* (London, 1958). p. 102.
[35] op. cit., pp. 102–3.

freedom from all constricting influences which overtakes a man when he finds he can lay aside the body, and when he discovers his inherent freedom and the immensity of space being his for the exploring. Such experiences are, however, within the realm of *prakṛti* or *māyā* and therefore can give but an inkling of what the supreme bliss (*parama-ānanda*) of the Self realisation may be, but they are experiences attested to by other people besides yogins, shamans, etc., all corroborating the truth as to the feeling of immense joy.[36]

IV *antarikṣeṇa patati viśvā rūpā-ava cākāśat,*
munir devasya-devasya saukṛtyāya sakhā hitaḥ.

Through the middle region flies the sage shining down upon all forms; for his piety is he deemed the friend of every god.

The fourth stanza has its counterpart in the first half of *Atharvaveda* VI.180.1, where the heavenly 'dog' is depicted in almost the same words: 'He flies through the atmosphere, looking down upon all things (*bhūtas*).'

The word *antarikṣa* corroborates our previous reading and emphasises the fact that the experiences mentioned are pertaining to the lower levels of the cosmos in its subtle aspect. The etymology gives out its meaning perfectly clearly: 'that which is seen within, *i.e.* not with the physical eyes' (*antar-īkṣa*) or 'that which dwells within' (*antari-kṣa*). It is usually translated by 'mid-air', 'middle-region', 'atmosphere' or 'sky' for want of understanding its intrinsic meaning. Aurobindo explains it as 'the intermediate, dynamic, vital or nervous consciousness' which corresponds to the subtle plane of cosmic existence, that realm which lies between the physical universe and the highest spiritual regions.

The *Ṛgveda* divides the world into two realms, heaven and earth, but this is a broad generalisation. When the *ṛṣis* want to be more specific, then we find three realms of cosmic existence being described, each susceptible of further division. These three main spheres have

[36] *Vide* R. C. Johnson, *The Imprisoned Splendour* (London, 1953), pp. 218–40. S. J. Muldoon and H. Carrington, *The Projection of the Astral Body* (London, 1929). R. Crookall, *The Study and Practice of Astral Projection: Analyses of Case Histories* (London, 1961).

frequently been taken in a strict physical sense by Western commentators: as the earth, the air, the sky. This, however, is fundamentally incorrect or else an extremely crude version of what the modern seer-philosopher and *Ṛgveda* interpreter Aurobindo perceived. Earth or *pṛthivī*, as already explained, refers to the mundane sphere or physical existence, the grossest form of the cosmos. *Antarikṣa* thus does not refer to the atmosphere, which is but a form of physical existence, it is rather that dimension of the subtle (*sūkṣma*) cosmos which is closest to the physical world. The third division implying the uppermost regions of the subtle or spiritual cosmos is called *dyu*, with *svar* as the highest 'heaven'. These divisions, barely outlined here, may nevertheless give us some hints as to the meaning of the 'six realms' or *rajāṃsi* of the *Ṛgveda*, the 'six burthens',[37] the 'three earths'[38] and the 'thrice three habitations' of the gods.[39]

The *muni* flies through the 'middle region', and his radiance is so strong that it seems to envelop all forms with its lustre. The verb *kāśate*, of which the intensive form is here used, has two meanings: 'to be visible, to appear' and 'to shine on' or 'be brilliant'; coupled with *ava*, it conveys the idea of looking or shining down upon. The word *rūpa* ('form') obviously implies all manifested things of the physical universe, animate and inanimate. One of the most significant characteristics of the intermediate sphere, also referred to as astral world, is stated to be its radiance and brightness. The *muni* who has left his physical body and is roaming about in this luminous region, in a body composed of subtle matter of the same brilliance as the surrounding 'ether', may well have the impression of casting 'light' down upon the 'shadows' of the physical cosmos. His ability to move freely in this bright realm makes him equal to the 'shining ones', the gods. Furthermore, through his pious deeds he is deemed the friend of every god. We are not told what kind of pious deeds (*saukṛtya*) the *muni* performs, but we are indirectly made to understand that because of these he is as holy as any god. The word *saukṛtya* may simply refer to his performance of ascetic practices, but on the other hand it could hint at the commonplace that no one can be a *muni* unless he has developed the moral qualities to the highest, for the gods of whom he is said to be a friend and to whom he is compared in point of goodness were, in Vedic

[37] Ṛgv. III.56.2.
[38] Ṛgv. VII.104.11.
[39] Ṛgv. III.56.5.

times, the agents of cosmic harmony, *ṛta*, the overseers of the statutes of divine law.

> v *vātasya-aśvo vāyoḥ sakhā-atho deveṣito muniḥ,*
> *ubhau samudrāv ā kṣeti yaś ca pūrva uta-aparaḥ.*
>
> The wind's steed, the Lord of life's friend, is the god-intoxicated sage; within both oceans he dwells, the upper and the lower.

Vāyu is now mentioned for the first time, and we have both *vāta* and *vāyu* brought close together. The 'wind's steed' and the 'breath-of-life's companion', or as translated above, are descriptive epithets which call for deeper consideration than has so far been accorded them in connection with the wind.

Aurobindo, in the Vedic Glossary compiled by A. B. Purani, has this to say: 'In the Vedic system Vāyu is the Master of Life, inspirer of that breath or dynamic energy called prāṇa which is represented in man by the vital or nervous activity. Vāyu is always associated with the prāṇa or life-energy.'[40] One may indeed wonder whether Vāyu was not at one time the personification of that breath (Hebrew *nephesh* as against *ruach*, the soul) which in Genesis God breathed into Adam to make him into a living being. Breath is not the spirit in the highest sense, that is the Self, rather it may be one of its lowest manifestations. Aurobindo furthermore states: 'By the ancient mystics life was considered to be a great force pervading all material existence. . . . It is this idea that was formulated later on in the conception of the prāṇa, the universal breath of life. All the vital and nervous activities of the human being fall within the definition of prāṇa, and belong to the domain of Vāyu.'[41] From the breath of the primeval man (*puruṣa*), Vāyu was born, declares the famous *puruṣa-sūkta* of the *Ṛgveda*. This expresses his high importance better than any commentary. In the *Atharvaveda* we find a whole panegyric for *prāṇa* in the hymn XI.4 of which the fifteenth verse shows *prāṇa* identified with the wind: 'Breath they call Mātariśvan; breath is called the wind; in breath what has been and what will be, in breath is all established.'

[40] A. B. Purani, *Śrī Aurobindo's Vedic Glossary* (Pondicherry, 1962), p. 82.
[41] Aurobindo, *On the Veda* (Pondicherry, 1964), p. 323.

M. Eliade gives an excellent summing up: 'The "breaths" . . . were identified with the cosmic winds [*Ath. Veda* XI.4.15], and with the cardinal points [*Chāndogya-Up*. III.13.1–5]. Air "weaves" the universe [*Bṛhadāraṇyaka-Up*. III.7.2], and breath "weaves" man [*Ath. Veda* X.2.13], and this symbolism of weaving developed in India into the grandiose concept of cosmic illusion, Māyā. . . .'[42]

Monier-Williams furthermore, in his standard dictionary, comments upon the fact that Vāyu 'is often made to occupy the same chariot with Indra, and in conjunction with him honoured with the first draught of the soma libation'.[43] The close connection of the two is quite striking throughout the *Ṛgveda*. One could speculate here *ad libitum* about the parallel which exists at the physical level between thought and breath. When thought stops, breath stops or becomes so shallow as to virtually stop. Both seem to be two lines of activity going on in very close conjunction. Indra viewed from the symbolical standpoint represents the 'great' (*mahat*) macrocosmically and *manas* microcosmically. Aurobindo yet again has a meaningful comment in this respect: '. . . for man it is the meeting of life with Mind and the support given by the former to the evolution of the latter which is the important aspect of Vāyu'.[44]

One may well wonder whether the *muni's* companionship with Vāyu, as expressed in the fifth stanza, is not a way of hinting at his perfect mastery over *prāṇa*, an achievement which would bring these early ascetics in direct line with the later yogins. The hymn, as should be obvious by now, proceeds by allusions, so that it is possible to indulge in various surmises. For M. Eliade 'the references to the horse of the wind, to the poison that he drinks with Rudra, to the gods whom he incarnates point rather to a shamanizing technique'.[45] Nevertheless, it may not be fruitless to examine the Yogic technique of controlling the currents of *prāṇa* in this connection.

To the yogin, who may well be compared to a surgeon, *prāṇa* is like a knife which he carefully employs to operate on his own mind, to cut out the malicious thoughts and feelings in order to pierce through to higher levels of consciousness.[46] In the strictest sense, *prāṇa* is not mere breath, although the two are closely knit. It is more akin to vital force

[42] M. Eliade, *Yoga: Immortality and Freedom*, p. 235.
[43] Monier-Williams' Sanskrit dictionary, p. 904.
[44] Aurobindo, *On the Veda*, p. 324.
[45] M. Eliade, *Yoga: Immortality and Freedom*, p. 102.
[46] We are indebted for this simile to Professor H. Upadhyay.

or life energy which we constantly inhale as we breathe in, which pervades our constitution and is life itself: the complete withdrawal of *prāṇa* from the body means death. This must have been known to the *ṛṣis* of Ṛgvedic India.[47]

Starting from the physical basis, by means of regulation, control and restraint (*āyāma*) of *prāṇa*, the yogin first gains mastery over the *prāṇa* currents, then over his body, arouses the *kuṇḍalinī*[48] or serpent fire and, by directing its course, activates the various vital centres (*cakras*) and finally forces the *kuṇḍalinī* to the crown centre, the abode of the Absolute. As in any other form of Yoga, the whole process ends with the realisation of the Self, the union of the transcendent, Śiva, and its power aspect, *śakti*. The science of *prāṇāyāma* is most intimately connected with the secret of *kuṇḍalinī*, hence with the 'inner heat', and it seems very likely that the term *tapas* covered, in Ṛgvedic times, aspects of this science. The descriptive epithets *vātasya aśvo*, *vāyoḥ sakhā* and, above all, *agniṃ bibharti* seem to be a perfect and pithy metaphoric image of a master of *prāṇa* and of fire. The whole hymn, with its emphasis upon the conquest of the two worlds, the evident feeling at home in the intermediate realm, point to an achievement for which a technique must surely have been devised already in those early days. That there is no specific mention of it in the *Ṛgveda* proves nothing. The words *agniṃ bibharti* suffice to point to such a knowledge. Even if not as detailed and assured as it developed in due time, such a technique may nevertheless have anticipated the later Yogic practices. The resemblances, so far as they can be worked out through the allusions, between these early *munis* and the yogins of historic times are too striking to be dismissed. Yet no clue is actually given in any of the stanzas as to how the *muni* did acquire his powers, whether by strict and stern self-discipline alone, by sheer practices similar to those described above, by performing certain rites or by adhering to specific orgiastic cults, as some would believe. However, Eliade has a further

[47] A hint given in Ṛgv. I.66.1, for example, seems to point this out: 'Like the sun's glance, like breath which is life (*āyur na prāṇo*).' The Sanskrit here has simply the equation of breath with life; like life-breath.

[48] The word from the adjective *kuṇḍalin* meaning 'circular' and as a substantive *kuṇḍalī* ('snake') could be traced to (1) the verbal root *kuṇḍ* ('to burn'), (2) *kuṇḍa* ('bowl, hole') or (3) *kuṇḍala* ('ring, coil of a rope'). From these one gathers the essential meaning: the fiery power coiled serpent-like in the bowl, the lotus or *cakra* at the base of the spine. *Cf.* 'Agni, Atharvan drew thee forth from the lotus flower by rubbing.' (Ṛgv. VI.16.13.).

interesting comment which elucidates the whole question a little more:

> On the plane of mystical technique in the strict sense, the most striking similarity between shamanism and yoga is represented by the production of 'inner heat'. We have shown that this is a universally disseminated technique . . . that this . . . is connected with the 'mastery of fire', a feat of fakirdom that must be regarded as the most archaic element of the magical tradition. We may conclude that from its earliest beginnings yoga knew the production of inner heat by retention of breath. For *tapas* is already attested in the Vedic period, and respiratory discipline was practised by the mysterious ecstatics knowns as *vrātyas*.[49]

For M. Bloomfield 'Who but Sūrya is "the horse of the wind, the companion of Vāyu, the *muni*, urged on his course by the gods, who lives in both seas, the eastern and the western"? . . . Therefore Sūrya is also the subject of stanza 5 . . . "He flies through the air looking upon all beings, he the *muni*, the friend good to benefit every god"'.[50] 'The word *avacākaśat* "looking at" is', he goes on, 'otherwise applied to the sun at AV. XIII.2.12 . . . XIII.4.1.'[51] The argument here shows complete ignorance of Yogic processes. For Bloomfield the fifth stanza of *Ṛgveda* X.136 is comparable to *Atharvaveda* XI.5.6 both of which he considers 'peculiarly suggestive of the sun'.[52] We can see but an extreme similarity with *Ṛgveda* X.136.5 and its description of the *muni*, but do not find any reference to the sun:

> The Brahmacārin advances, kindled by the firewood, clothed in the skin of the black antelope, consecrated, with long beard. Within the day he passes from the eastern to the northern sea; gathering together the worlds he repeatedly shapes them.[53]

The last two phrases may have given rise to this misunderstanding, but they may bear a different connotation. The sun may be considered

[49] M. Eliade, *Yoga: Immortality and Freedom*, p. 337.
[50] M. Bloomfield, 'Contributions to the interpretation of the Veda. II: The two dogs of Yama in a new role', p. 167.
[51] op. cit., p. 168.
[52] M. Bloomfield, *Hymns of the Atharvaveda*, Sacred Books of the East, vol. XLII (1897), p. 627.
[53] op. cit., p. 215.

the heavenly ascetic wandering from East to West and hence the prototype of the *muni* described here, but the details of the hymn apply to human beings rather than the sun.

The sage, divinely impelled (*deveṣitaḥ*),[54] translated here 'god-intoxicated', is obviously inspired by the gods. Only two specific gods are mentioned, Vāyu of whom Vāta is the *alter ego* and Rudra, the other entities, *gandharvas* and *apsaras* not being *devas*. But it may be surmised that the sage keeps company with any of the gods, since he has found entrance into their domains and, alternatively, has let them pervade his whole being. He dwells upon or in both oceans. The words which qualify these, *pūrva* and *uta-apara*, are usually translated as 'Eastern' and 'Western'. However, the primary meaning of these words is 'upper' and 'lower'. As the sage has already been referred to in the first stanza as having mastery over the two worlds, mind and matter, this particular verse may be only another reference to these two realms, the higher and the lower, the spiritual and the physical. The *muni* is at ease in both spheres, since he is master of life. This seems to be far more in the spirit of the hymn than any particular moving whether of the *muni* or of the sun from a physical Eastern to a Western ocean, or *vice versa*. Indeed, we fail to see the point of such a reference, unless it means that there are *munis* everywhere, a particularly meaningless statement, or once again, unless the East and the West are taken in the ancient sense of the realm of light and darkness, life and death, an interpretation which joins our original view, for the abode of the living and of the dead is precisely the physical and the supraphysical or spiritual world respectively. The word *samudra* is thus explained in Aurobindo's glossary: 'We notice first that existence itself is constantly spoken of in Hindu writings . . . and even philosophical reasoning and illustration as an ocean. The Veda speaks of two oceans, the upper and lower waters, the supraconscient and the subconscient oceans.'[55] We cannot dismiss the 'psychic' or psychological interpretation, as L. Renou was inclined to do, particularly in connection with this hymn, the precursor of Yogic psychology.

VI *apsarasāṃ gandharvāṇām mṛgāṇāṃ caraṇe caran,*
keśī ketasya vidvānt sakhā svādur madintamaḥ.

[54] Derived from √*iṣ*, 'to move', and therefore 'to be driven, animated, excited'.
[55] A. B. Purani, *Śrī Aurobindo's Vedic Glossary*, p. 93.

> In the path of nymphs, angels, wild beasts wanders the long-haired one, the knower of heart's desire, a gentle friend, most exhilarating.

Further details about the *muni's* free wanderings are now given. During these he encounters three kinds of creatures: the *apsaras*, the *gandharvas* and the *mṛgas*. The first two classes are not denizens of the physical plane, but the third class belongs to it, unless perhaps the term *mṛga* refers to some wild beast known to Indian mythology. If not, there may be a deliberate mixing up of the planes of consciousness, perhaps to emphasise the fact that the *muni* is at home on both. Sāyaṇa interprets this first part of the verse as 'in heaven, in the air and on earth'. This would make the *apsaras* the inhabitants of the upper spiritual and the *gandharvas* of the lower spiritual or intermediate world, whereas both belong rather together and perhaps more to the latter than the former. Taking into consideration the third or physical cosmos first, the *muni* wanders unharmed amidst the wild beasts. This is a fact well attested to this day; no animal, however wild or fierce, will ever attack a holy man, who can roam in and out of the jungle, quite unaware of his surroundings, in perfect safety. As the *Yoga-Sūtra* states: '[When the yogin] is grounded in [the practice of] non-harming (*ahiṃsā*), his presence [effects] the abandonment of hostility [in others].'[56]

The *apsaras* and *gandharvas*, who figure prominently in Indian mythology, are certainly no earthly creatures. In trying to find an equivalent term or idea in the English language and European lore we had to fall back upon 'nymphs' and 'angels' to translate each respectively, although 'nymph' does not convey quite the same notion as *apsarā*. The *apsaras* were supposed to be the wives of the *gandharvas*. This is clearly stated in the *Atharvaveda*, from which it is easy to conclude that they were simply the feminine counterpart of the *gandharvas*. These are mentioned several times in the *Ṛgveda*, usually in the singular. They are not considered *devas* although their functions, in some respects, are similar to the latter's. Far more than the *devas*, they elude attempts at understanding their specific being.

H. W. Wallis points out that the use of the plural for the *gandharva* in the *Ṛgveda* is very rare, and cites but one example, apart from X.136, namely IX.113.2 from which he concludes that the *Ṛgveda*

[56] YS II.35: *ahiṃsā-pratiṣṭhāyāṃ tat-saṃnidhau vaira-tyāgaḥ.*

recognises one *gandharva* only.[57] The word, however, is also used in the plural in *Ṛgveda* III.38.6 and this use, although restricted, does point to a knowledge of more than one. It may be that the early Vedic people believed in one tutelary or guardian angel who was in close contact with their *devas*, whilst recognising that there were others who did not concern themselves with human beings. We do not accept Wallis' opinion that 'the conception of the rising sun in the morning dew is personified in the figure of the Gandharva'.[58] This is a typical example of the Western scholar trying at all costs to find a physical phenomenon to account for something which is essentially spiritual or supraphysical.

The *gandharvas* of the Vedic *saṃhitās*, the angels of biblical cosmogony, are, according to the testimony of the yogins and mystics, living entities from the centre of whose being radiate effulgent streams of force or light perceptible to man only when he is in a certain state of ecstasy. Hence the similar descriptions, Vedic and biblical, which would repay a deeper study. The rainbow (Grassmann's interpretation), the solar beams (Griffith's suggestion), are but attempts to reduce to physical terms what eludes the senses and the intellect. In this respect, the description of the angel found in Revelation is of interest:

> And I saw another mighty angel come down from heaven, clothed with a cloud: and a rainbow was upon his head, and his face was as it were the sun, and his feet as pillars of fire.[59]

Similarly Ezekiel's vision as recounted by the prophet himself in the Old Testament would lead to further insights, but one interesting point ought to be mentioned here: the beams or flashes of force or light radiating from these entities are taken for wings without any questioning in the Hebrew and Christian scriptures, or occasionally as wheels, a fine example of how the human mind automatically shapes into something known what it encounters as fundamentally formless and elusive. In the *Ṛgveda*, on the other hand, these luminous flashes are described as hair, long flowing hair, an epithet also applied to Agni and Sūrya. So we have the *gandharva* 'whose hair is borne upon the wind'.[60] That the angel belongs to the spiritual realm and not to the physical is

[57] H. W. Wallis, *The Cosmology of the Ṛgveda* (London, 1887), pp. 75–6.
[58] op. cit., p. 34.
[59] New Testament, Revelation X.1.
[60] Ṛgv. III.38.6.

confirmed in the following verse: 'There saw I, going thither in the mind, *gandharvas* in their course.'[61] The very fact of 'going thither in the mind (*manasā*)' militates against Griffith's awkward suggestion that the *gandharvas* are 'probably . . . merely sunbeams'. These entities can be met with only in their own realms to which the *munis* have gained access, and to these, as to the *ṛṣis*, they impart 'in the spirit' (*manasā*) heavenly secrets and inspire the thoughts or visions (*dhiya*) of mortals who pray and make offerings to them.[62] The possibility of contacting supraphysical beings is also pointed out by Patañjali who, however, warns the yogin not to pride himself on this achievement: 'When [the adept] is invited by higher beings (*sthānins*), there should arise no attachment or pride [in him], for [he would only come] into renewed contact with the undesired [suffering and bondage to the world].'[63]

The *munis* have also gained entrance into the human heart: *keśī ketasya vidvān*. The word *keta*, variously translated and interpreted, points to a power of the ascetic on which Patañjali makes some useful observations. He explains the possibility of knowing the mind of others through the practice of *saṃyama* ('constraint'), that is concentration, meditation and enstasis upon one and the same object. The following aphorism is particularly relevant: '[By *saṃyama*] upon the awarenesses [there arises] knowledge of the mind of others.'[64] Furthermore he states: '[By *saṃyama*] upon the heart [there arises] understanding (*saṃvit*) of the [own] mind.'[65] Such a knowledge of the heart's desire makes the *muni* the most understanding, sympathetic of friends, a gentle (*svādu*), most exhilarating (*madintama*) friend who reaches out to all, his own exhilaration being communicated to all those with whom he comes into contact.

VII *vāyur asmā upa-amanthat pinaṣṭi smā kunamnamā,*
keśī viṣasya pātreṇa yad rudreṇa-apibat saha.

For him has the Lord of life churned and pounded the unbendable, when the long-haired one in Rudra's company drank from the poison cup.

[61] Ṛgv. III.38.6.
[62] *Vide* Ṛgv. X.139.5.
[63] YS III.51: *sthāny-upanimantraṇe saṅga-smaya-akaraṇaṃ punar-aniṣṭa-prasaṅgāt.*
[64] YS III.19: *pratyayasya para-citta-jñānam.*
[65] YS III.34: *hṛdaye citta-saṃvit.*

This is the most enigmatic of all the stanzas. It certainly points to the close connection between Rudra and the *keśins* and may lend weight to the argument that the latter, with Rudra as their tutelar deity, represent a different line of culture or worship from that of the *ṛṣis*. Here is a clear statement that in the company of the god Rudra, the *keśins*, who are not deified, take their place to partake of a specific drink. But we cannot at all agree with H. D. Griswold's remark about these *keśins* 'drinking poison-liquids that produce ecstasy'.[66]

R. N. Dandekar asserts concerning *Ṛgveda* X.136: 'This hymn clearly relates to the specific orgiastic cult of the *munis*. These . . . seem to have . . . indulged in a sort of ecstasy-producing medicament (X.136.7). There are also indications that they attained certain miraculous or mystic powers which are comparable to the powers which are believed to be attained through *yoga*. Rudra is represented in this *muni-sūkta* almost as the leader of that cult.'[67] The reference to the orgiastic cult is probably based upon the poison quaffing, but the latter is no proof of this.

The pedigree of Rudra so far remains more or less a mystery. R. N. Dandekar and V. G. Rahurkar argue that he was indigenous to pre-Vedic India. It is indeed noticeable that he plays little part in Vedic rituals. Rudra is not one of the Adityas who are invited to sit on the sacrificial grass for the purely orthodox rites. Dandekar observes that he did play his part in the purely popular ceremonies.[68] From this we have to conclude that he was only later on assimilated to the Vedic pantheon. This yet again draws a line of difference between the *ṛṣis* and the *munis* and would indicate two separate cults. In the *Ṛgveda*, Rudra is identified with Agni: 'Thou, Agni, art Rudra, the deity of the great sky.'[69] The same is found in the *Atharvaveda* (VIII.87.1), the *Śatapatha-Brāhmaṇa* (VI.1.3.10) and the *Taittirīya-Brāhmaṇa* (II.2.2.3). Are we to conclude from this that Rudra was accepted into the Vedic pantheon via his likeness to Agni, or was he just another name used by different tribes for a conception similar to that personified in Agni—the creator, and the destroyer, the beneficent and the maleficent, the healer and the killer?

[66] H. D. Griswold, *The Religion of the Ṛgveda* (London, 1923), p. 339.

[67] R. N. Dandekar, 'Rudra in the Veda', *Journal of the University of Poona*, I (1953), p. 99.

[68] op. cit., p. 98.

[69] Ṛgv. II.1.6.

In the essay on *Ṛgveda* X.129, we have tried to show that the roots of the Sāṃkhya ontology can be traced back to Ṛgvedic times as basic, still hardly outlined ideas. The enigmatic phrase 'Vāyu (the master of *prāṇa*) churns or stirs up and pounds or grinds the unbendable (*kunamnamā*)' appears to refer to the action of *prāṇa* upon the body, the key words here being 'stir up' (*amanthat*) and 'grind' (*pinaṣṭi*) expressing the action that is being performed upon the unbendable which may be identified with *tamas*, one of the three primary energies of *prakṛti*: *tamas* or inertia, heaviness, the gross aspect, the mass-stuff, that which provides the necessary resistance and hence the resulting friction without which no step, no action could be taken, but which, at the same time, must be made malleable or pliable, must be bent to a mere tool or stepping-stone in the hands of the yogin, in order that finally harmony or *sattva* may prevail. Inertia, darkness (*tamas*), man's material nature, thus stands as a mountain rock or inflexible basis which nevertheless is to be bent if the yogin will achieve his purpose. When *tamas* has been subdued, there is created a proper climate wherein the *kuṇḍalinī* can be stirred up and made to rise, eventually to illuminate the whole being. By the grace of the Lord, in this case Rudra, with the help of Vāyu, the *muni* was able to achieve self-conquest. As a result the poison of the world could have no effect upon him, and like any god he could even drink of it.

This drinking of poison, in one of its connotations, is closely associated with the original churning of the ocean which, in its mythological significance, takes us back to cosmogenesis: the extracting out of the vast upheaval, out of the churning, stirring, moulding, shattering and refashioning, of the world, the essence or nectar of immortality, the goal of this stupendous process. Through life in the ocean of matter the *devas* obtained the immortal beverage. One may speculate that before the mortal may absorb the strong ambrosia which the gods hold out to him, the poison thrown off like foam from the ocean waves must be drunk; yet only those who have achieved a measure of control over themselves can do so consciously without ill effects, the others must bide their time and let themselves be tossed by the waves of matter until they too have learnt to steer their bark safely and can drink their full cup. Hence the warning:

Let no one other than a superior being ever even in thought practise the same [the daring acts superior beings perform]; any one who through folly does so, perishes, like anyone not a Rudra [drinking] the poison produced from the ocean.[70]

J. Muir explains this verse as referring 'to the poison drunk by Śiva at the churning of the ocean'. That the *muni* is shown drinking with Rudra must be an allusion to his having achieved complete self-mastery, hence godhood. Surely, *viṣa* in this context means more than water. The final question must be: has such a drinking any symbolic reference to a taking upon oneself of the sins of mankind? This would be quite in keeping with Indian tradition, but was the idea already prevalent in Vedic times? If holy men had already reached great heights of spiritual consciousness, then the meaning of self-sacrifice, indeed of bare 'sacrifice', could not have been alien to them. Vedic cosmogenesis is based upon the original divine sacrifice and the sacrificial rituals were instituted as a perpetual reminder of this universal phenomenon. A. Ch. Bose makes the following comment: 'The Vedic muni makes the supreme sacrifice not only by courting death in the service of the world but also by taking the world's sufferings on himself—drinking from the poison cup in Rudra's company.'[71] This strikes a slightly dramatic note not quite in keeping with the Indian spirit for whom tragedy has no place. Does the *muni* accept the cup of water of life or poison from the hands of Rudra—another reference to his bearing the two worlds—that he may be a light unto all men?—All these points arise in the course of examining these age-old myths, but they cannot at present be fully answered.

The human mind has somewhat changed during the last few thousands of years and now views in a different light what it formerly expressed as myth. Yet, fundamentally, the great truths remain the same. The sage of every age still accepts or takes upon himself the sins or sufferings of others that he might alleviate the karma of the world. The path to Self-realisation is still the path of discipline, one-pointedness in word, deed and thought.

[70] *Bhagavata-Purāṇa* X.33.31. The translation is that of J. Muir.
[71] A. Ch. Bose, *Hymns from the Vedas* (London, 1966), p. 157.

6 *The Heart of Ṛgvedic Religion: Agni, Flame Divine*

Agni am I who know, by birth, all
creatures . . . I am light threefold,
measurer of the region.[1]

Agni, the flame divine, the life blood of the universe, the mighty force at work within all things, is the most dynamic and enigmatic of Vedic deities. *Flame of warmth* that builds up the cosmos—that force which whirls the atoms and molecules, and in this whirling moulds the substances and shapes the forms life assumes in its eternal activities; *flame of destruction* that shatters all worn out forms, that ruthless power which made the poet lament of nature red in tooth and claw, forgetting that life itself is never destroyed, but only its habitations, that new, more perfected ones may find expression; *flame of purification* urging all things onwards and driving man on to the pinnacles of human achievement; *flame of love* the foundation, love the ultimate! Such is Agni, the beloved god, the many-sided power, benevolent and dangerous, mysterious in his workings, far-reaching in his activities, sublime in his lofty sweeps, the most concrete and the most abstract Vedic deity, the very expression of the divine will made manifest through the cosmos. The Vedic seers were so struck by him that they composed some of their most beautiful hymns in his honour, and in the *Ṛgveda* gave him pride of place.

Why was fire, and fire alone out of all the elements, chosen throughout the ages and by different races at different epochs as the best capable of representing, to the human mind, the dynamic aspect of deity?[2] For this is exactly what Agni represents. Water, out of the

[1] Ṛgv. III.26.7.

[2] 'This world order, the same for all beings, neither any of the gods hath made nor any man; but it always was, is and shall be, ever-living fire, kindled in measure and quenched in measure.' (Heracleitus, Fragment D. 30.)

elements, was selected to express matter or the great nurturing mother of the universe, through whom and in whom life's seed is brought to birth and fruition, that seed being also Agni. Furthermore, fire has even been boldly equated with deity by all the ancients, including those who cannot be 'accused' of being fire-worshippers, as in the following Hebrew statement: 'The Lord is a consuming fire.'[3] It is a fact that all religions, whether Vedic, Parsi, Hebrew, Christian, even Muslim, have expressed the divine impact upon man's nature in terms of fire. So also has the manifestation of deity upon earth been thus depicted. The three following examples from the Old Testament might suffice to illustrate the point: 'And Mount Sinai was altogether on a smoke, because the Lord descended upon it in fire.'[4] It could be added here that only Moses could stand this fire face to face, but had to veil his own face which radiated so strongly when he turned back to the common people lest the effulgence should make them flee in terror. 'And the sight of the glory of the Lord was like devouring fire on the top of the mount in the eyes of the children of Israel.'[5] The prophet Elijah was taken up to heaven in a glory of fire: 'Behold, there appeared a chariot of fire and horses of fire . . . and Elijah went up by a whirlwind into heaven.'[6] So also, we might recall how in the New Testament the Holy Spirit manifested as cloven tongues of fire settling upon each apostle at Pentecost and illuminating each one with divine light.

At first glance, to understand the why of this particular equation of fire and deity may appear rather difficult. But there is behind this a deep spiritual experience and a great knowledge which, when grasped, yields a key to the significance of the many-sidedness of Agni, indeed to the mystery of fire itself, to its elevation throughout antiquity to the perfect manifestation of the spiritual. Was the Vedic *ṛṣi*, it may be asked, when he invoked Agni—the messenger of gods and men, the sacrificial priest—fully aware of all the implications latent in the meaning of fire? The descriptive epithets lavished upon Agni and the many cryptic statements and references made to his various aspects do point to a complete science underlying the invocations, the praises, the exaltations, a science which bears the deepest scrutiny, but has been left unfathomed by Western exegesis.

[3] Deuteronomy IV.24.
[4] Exodus XIX.8.
[5] Exodus XXIV.17.
[6] Second Book of Kings II.11.

Vedic literature refers to three 'types' of fire. This differentiation is already apparent in the *Ṛgveda*, and it may be expressed, as Western scholars following Indian commentators have done, as *fire by friction, solar fire* and *electric fire*—the lightning fire—without, however, subscribing to the purely literal interpretation so characteristic of the West; for each type of fire may have its physical, literal meaning, but certainly also has its symbolic, spiritual significance. The three fires are viewed as 'the ramifications of Agni' (Ṛgv. I.59.1).[7] The *Bṛhaddevatā*, a contribution to the meaning of the deities and mysteries of the *Ṛgveda*, attributed to Śaunaka, divides the three thus: 'Agni in this [world], Indra and Vāyu in the middle, Sūrya in heaven, are here to be recognised as the three deities.'[8] So also the same significant division is met with in the *Viṣṇu-Purāṇa* (IV.6). Agni himself states unequivocably: 'I am light threefold.' (Ṛgv. III.26.7) There is thus constant emphasis upon the 'threefold essence' which is also represented as the handiwork of the gods.[9]

Agni has three 'births' (Ṛgv. IV.1.7) and abodes: in heaven, on earth, in the waters or air's mid-region (*antarikṣa*); that is, in the spiritual, the material and the intermediate realm, however this may be interpreted. At other times he is spoken of as the child of the 'two parents', the spiritual and the material, the primeval parents Heaven and Earth. At the highest level, Agni's birth lies in the divine 'desire' (*kāma*) for manifestation.[10] Thence, he is kindled to his dynamic fiery form through the interaction of the celestial parents, the positive and the negative, *dyu* and *pṛthivī* (*puruṣa* and *prakṛti* in later terminology), 'when unfurled the mighty billows that generated the universal matrix conceiving fire' (Ṛgv. X.121.7). Agni is propelled outwards on his cosmic task of creation to burst forth upon every rung of the ladder of life, to be conceived by the gods themselves and through them as a gift to mankind, finally by man himself—'he, Agni, *whom the gods have generated*, in whom they offered up all worlds and creatures' (Ṛgv. X.88.9). One is tempted here to use an expression

[7] The word *vayā*, translated by 'ramification', has the meaning of strength, power, then of branch, twig, then of race, family. From these we can conclude that the three fires are the expressions, the powers of Agni as manifested on three distinct levels.

[8] *Bṛhaddevatā* I.69.

[9] *Vide* Ṛgv. X.88.10.

[10] *Vide* Ṛgv. X.129.4.

from the field of electricity: the gods are really stepping down, from unmanifested cosmic realms, the effulgent dynamic power which is both destructive and constructive. Moreover, Agni, dormant in undeveloped man, links 'heaven' and 'earth' in awakened man. So the following cryptic verse is pregnant with meaning: 'Forehead of the sky, earth's centre, Agni became the messenger of Earth and Heaven.'[11] Thereby he unites the opposite poles which originally he had 'spread out' by his 'power' (*kratu*),[12] his dominion exerting itself in the three realms of manifestation. 'He has laid down his vital germ within these worlds.'[13] The following enigmatic verses should now become intelligible: 'Child of a double birth he grasps at triple food.'[14] And: 'He, doubly born, hath spread in his effulgence through the three luminous realms, through all the regions.'[15] Within man he brings the two poles together, for he raises the merely human or mortal to the immortal. Even so, he is 'the wise son of heaven and the child of earth' (III.25.1.). Hence he is 'the mighty one whose power extends over the two worlds' (*dvibarhā mahi*).[16] Yet again the meaning of the three births is given from a different aspect: 'First Agni sprang to life from out of Heaven; the second time from us came the knower of births; thirdly the manly-souled was in the waters.'[17]

Spiritual (heaven), human (with the emphasis upon the mental) and material, the three aspects are united as one in Agni. The seers 'know' Agni's 'three powers in three stations'—'We know thy forms in many a place divided. We know what name supreme thou hast in secret. We know the source from which thou hast proceeded' (X.45.2). This is as full an admission as could be given by any seer as to his secret knowledge. It could not have been merely the physical fire that alerted the *ṛṣis* to the reality of a spiritual flame present in nature, man and deity, but a 'vision' (*dhī*) of an inner reality, and also, one may conjecture, their 'seeing' within themselves the upward rising flame of which the Tantric *kuṇḍalinī*, the serpent fire coiled at rest in the *mūlādhāra-cakra*, is the physical, though subtle counterpart. This

[11] Ṛgv. I.59.2.
[12] *Vide* Ṛgv. III.6.5.
[13] Ṛgv. III.2.10.
[14] Ṛgv. I.140.2.
[15] Ṛgv. I.149.4.
[16] Ṛgv. IV.5.3. The phrase *dvibarhā mahi* literally means 'mightily expanding in two places'.
[17] Ṛgv. X.45.1.

'dynamo', whether physical or spiritual, asleep in the average person, is when awakened as constructive or as destructive as fire—according to the motive that directs, is indeed fire.

There is no need to emphasise here the essential seership of the *ṛṣis*, the science of their meditation, thought, inspiration and vision and their constant referring to themselves as going or seeing 'in the spirit' or rather 'in the mind' (*manasā*) whatever they describe. The whole question has been thoroughly studied by J. Gonda,[18] and some aspects of it have been touched upon in the introductory notes.

The threefold division of fire should now be examined more closely.

1 *Earthly fire* or fire of nature, fire by friction, inherent in both the earth and every growth it bears, as also in man. The physical form of Agni is not merely what we see as flame, what flashes forth by the friction of two sticks, but that living principle, that warmth at the core of all things. This is brought out in many verses:

> He who grows mightily in herbs, within each
> fruitful mother and each babe she bears, wise,
> life of all men, in the waters' home.[19]

> He stirs with life in wombs dissimilar in kind,
> born as a lion or a loudly bellowing bull.[20]

So this flame-power that 'quickeneth the waters' seed' (Ṛgv. VIII.44.16) unites the macrocosm and the microcosm, nature and nature's child, man, in their essential being. One of the most superb hymns of the *Atharvaveda*, the hymn to Earth, shows this many-sidedness, yet underlying oneness of Agni so well understood in Vedic times:

> There lies the fire within the earth, and in
> plants, and waters carry it; the fire is in stone.
> There is a fire deep within men, a fire in the
> kine, and a fire in horses.

[18] *Vide* J. Gonda, *The Vision of the Vedic Poets* (The Hague, 1963).
[19] Ṛgv. I.67.5.
[20] Ṛgv. III.2.11.

The same fire that burns in the heavens;
the mid-air belongs to this Fire Divine.
Men kindle this fire that bears the oblation . . .[21]

The statement 'Agni, hidden, abiding in every wood' (Ṛgv. V.11.6) should now bear the light of a deeper interpretation than the mere literal one. If we remember that the word *vana* is also used in *Ṛgveda* X.81.4 and similar creation hymns, where it is asked 'from what wood was the universe produced' and may in these particular contexts be one of the many metaphors the poets delight in, and simply mean 'substance', we have a hint in *Ṛgveda* V.11.6 as in like verses of Agni's eternal presence in all things and of his action in all manifestation. 'Germ of the world, ensign of all creation' (Ṛgv. X.45.6) is he. Yet again: 'He who is germ of waters, germ of woods, germ of all things that move not and that move. . . . To him even in the rock and in the house . . .' (Ṛgv. I.70.2) *Garbha*, his seed or germ, is found in all things, animate and inanimate, for his is the fire that animates all substances, his the cosmic power at the root of all. Thanks to his hidden activity all things are brought out of the nurturing darkness of earth, where the seed may linger for long,[22] into the full light of day and maturity. As Śrī Aurobindo puts it: 'Agni's mission is . . . to raise up the soul struggling in nature from obscurity to the light.'[23] One senses here that a great plan is behind this constant quickening of creation, what in the *Ṛgveda* is obscurely referred to beneath the profound significance of Agni which this essay will endeavour to bring out: Agni's roaring, all-devouring and all-fostering and purifying life, a devouring which evokes far more of a sense of joy than dread; Agni 'the home to which the kine return, whom the fleet-foot coursers seek as home, and strong enduring steeds as home',[24] the meaning of which cannot be left at its face value, *i.e.* a physical fire lit up by humans to which the animals would come back at night possibly to sleep side by side with them. . . . Agni's home, the home of 'holy order' (*ṛta*),[25] which will be considered later on, is that hearth to which men are enjoined to lead all their ways,[26]

[21] *Ath. veda* XII.1.19,20. The translation is that of A. C. Bose, *Hymns from the Vedas* (London 1966).
[22] *Vide* Ṛgv. V.2.1,2.
[23] Aurobindo, *On the Veda* (Pondicherry, 1964), p. 401.
[24] Ṛgv. V.6.1.
[25] *Vide* Ṛgv. IV.1.12.
[26] *Vide* Ṛgv. I.66.5.

is that kindled god they wish to attain 'as cows their home at eve'; it is that heart of perfection towards which the whole creation strives. The Christian scriptures explained this idea, hardly outlined in the *Ṛgveda*, in terms of redemption, the bringing up of all forms to the perfect ideal held in the divine mind:

> For we know that the whole of creation is moaning in the pangs of childbirth until this hour until the creation itself would be set free from the thraldom of decay to enjoy the liberty that comes with the glory of the children of God.[27]

These two views, Vedic and Christian, dissimilar in their expression, fundamentally alike in their inner significance, could fruitfully be compared with what the advanced Western science has to offer in this respect:

> 'Men's minds are reluctant to recognise that evolution has a precise orientation and a privileged axis'. This is the cardinal postulate of the Teilhardian synthesis. Evolution, human and biological and cosmic, is not simply a lot of whirl and flutter going nowhere in particular . . . human evolution is an extension of biological evolution . . . man's ultimate concern, and his individual meaning and dignity are atoms of the meaning of the whole cosmos.[28]

II *Solar fire*: Agni, the 'finder of the light' (Ṛgv. III.26.1), is the fire in the sun—he is called upon as 'Savitṛ's productive power' (Ṛgv. VIII.91.6)—and therefore the life and light-giving principle present in the sun both as an actual physical fact and in a deeper sense as that inner light which, when kindled, gives enlightenment and meaning to existence. For the sun in the Vedic lore is not merely the beacon that lights up the sky and earth but also, and that is what above all is of interest, the inner light or sun of the human mental sky. Hence the following verses with their double meaning:

> Behold the rays of dawn, like heralds, lead on high the sun, that men may see the great all-knowing god. Beyond this lower gloom

[27] New Testament, Epistle to the Romans, VIII.16–24.
[28] T. Dobzhansky, *The Biology of Ultimate Concern* (London, 1967), p. 116.

> and upward to the light would we ascend O sun, thou god among the gods.[29]

> Looking upon the loftier light above the darkness, we have come to Sūrya, God among the gods, the light that is most excellent.[30]

Both sun and dawn seem to be treated at times as manifestations of Agni. In many instances, Agni is compared to the sun, more rarely identified with it:

> Like Sūrya with his fulgent rays, O Agni, thou overspreadest both the worlds with splendour.[31]

But there also are identifications as in *Ṛgveda* X.88.6 and 11 where Agni becomes Sūrya or manifests as Sūrya, this being a hint on the part of the seers as to the underlying oneness of all:

> Head of the world is Agni in the night time; then as the sun at morn springs up and rises.[32]

'The gods set Agni as Sūrya in heaven' (Ṛgv. X.88.11), here the sun is shown as an aspect, perhaps the more glorious aspect, of Agni and worshipped as such. In yet another verse he is the 'eye' (*cakṣus*) of Agni, as well as of Mitra and Varuṇa.[33] Many beautiful verses could be cited:

> In his arising Agni merges into the rays of the sun: touch the celestial summits with thy columns and overspread thee with the rays of Sūrya.[34]

> The soul of all that moveth not or moveth, the sun hath filled the air and earth and heaven.[35]

[29] Ṛgv. I.50.1.10. The translation is that of M. Monier-Williams, *Indian Wisdom* (London, 1893), p.17

[30] Ṛgv. I.50.10. Griffith's translation.

[31] Ṛgv. VI.4.6.

[32] Ṛgv. X.88.6.

[33] *Vide* Ṛgv. I.115.1.

[34] Ṛgv. VII.2.1.

[35] Ṛgv. I.115.1.

The latter quality of all-pervasiveness is most characteristic of Agni who is 'sunk in the lap of all that moves and moves not' (Ṛgv. I.146.1), of him 'whose active force is light' for his 'rays . . . through the nights glimmer sleepless, ageless, like the floods' (Ṛgv. I.143.3). There are thus affinities remarked between both, but not merely in the superficial, physical sense. Several enigmatic verses appear in a hymn addressed to Agni and point to the inner meaning of the sun and therefore of that aspect of the fire. The latter 'mid mortal men . . . is the light immortal' first sings the seer; then he goes on:

> A firm light (*dhruvaṃ jyotir*) hath been set for men to look on; among all things that fly the mind is swiftest . . . Mine ears unclose to hear, mine eye to see him; the light that harbours in my spirit broadens.[36]

This 'light' set for men to look on is comparable to the 'loftier light' (*jyotir-uttaram*) of *Ṛgveda* I.50.10. The poet, here as elsewhere, strives to behold or to express that deeper light whose flash illuminates the human mind and, like the sun or the flame divine, sets it ablaze; that light which is invoked in one of the most beautiful prayers the ancient Vedic world has handed down to us, recited to this day in all India:

> Let us meditate upon that celestial splendour of the solar lord. So may he inspire our prayers;[37]

that light of the sun which is also ascribed to the dead, that is, which is recognised as belonging to the 'fathers' as they have united themselves to the sun's beams.[38] How could the ancient fathers, the sages, be guardians of the sun, as stated in *Ṛgveda* X.154.5, in the beyond and give its light[39] except this light be of the spirit?

III *Electric fire*; the fire in the lightning flash, the power that smites down from heaven; the third aspect of Agni, considered here the most enigmatic, for it is only referred to by way of metaphors or enshrined in

[36] Ṛgv. VI.9.5,6.
[37] Ṛgv. III.62.10.
[38] *Vide* Ṛgv. I.109.7.
[39] *Vide* Ṛgv. X.107.1.

various myths or pictures, perhaps as an attempt to express, on the one hand, the purifying or punitive aspect of Agni, and on the other hand, that which in our innermost consciousness flashes forth and yet remains untouchable, unapproachable, which heralds a something beyond even consciousness, which heralds the dynamic lord of all creation. The present interpretation will be in opposition to that generally put forward by Western scholars and also will diverge considerably from orthodox Indian exegesis, especially in the order of treatment; for here, Agni's lightning aspect, because of its vast implications, is considered last and is not taken as being simply identified with Indra or Vāyu, but as being rooted beyond these. This, however, does not detract from the importance assigned to Sūrya who remains ever the light-giver in both the outer and inner meaning, an importance which in course of time was more and more emphasised by the Hindus. Only, the lightning side of Agni holds mysteries which still need to be probed.

> The thunderbolt often whirleth down from the lofty, misty realm of Sūrya. Beyond this realm there is another glory.[40]

The poet leaves this 'other glory' (*śravasḥ anya*) to our imagination or speculation. But the bolt that falls down from Sūrya's realm seems to take its root in the glory beyond even Sūrya, a conception that should be examined.

There is identity in essence between the earthly fire kindled upon the altar, or the quickening seed spurring all things to fruition, and the lightning that rends the firmament as well as the light-bringing sun, but each time the meteorological factor appears of little moment and is used as a poetic comparison, just as Agni (or Indra or Viṣṇu) is described as a 'bull'. Each metaphoric description, like car (*ratha*), lightning (*vidyut*), fire-hair (*śociṣkeśa*), has a specific meaning which should become clear in the course of this essay.[41] In the study of this lightning aspect of Agni, we come across certain myths evocative of man's dim past rich in most significant lore, a lore the deep meaning of

[40] Ṛgv. X.27.21.

[41] *Vide* Ṛgv. III.14.1: 'Agni the son of strength whose car is lightning, whose hair is flame.' Also Ṛgv. III.1.14: 'Like brilliant lightnings, mighty luminaries accompany the light-diffusing Agni.' Also Ṛgv. X.91.5: 'Thy glories are as lightnings from the rainy cloud . . . like heralds of the dawn's approach.'

which has been ignored to a large extent, except for one or two outstanding scholars, as for example Jean Herbert whose work in this connection is of the greatest importance. Agni's original birth is varied and depends upon the levels of manifestation on which he appears. With regard to the earthly level, he is specifically referred to as having been brought to men by Mātariśvan. Speculations have been rife as to the meaning of the latter. According to Śrī Aurobindo, the word 'seems to mean he who extends himself in the mother or the container, whether that be the containing mother element, Ether, or the material energy called Earth in the Veda'.[42] Etymologically the word is derived from *mātari*+*śvan* which itself comes from √*śvi* ('to swell, increase, grow'). As stated in the *Ṛgveda*, Agni when 'formed in his Mother is Mātariśvan; he hath, in his course, become the rapid flight of wind'.[43] Within the womb of matter develops the spark which then, like the wind that bloweth whither it listeth, manifests according to its wish. He appears then to be another presentation of Agni, both being often inextricably linked together. However, one may also assume that the name was given to one of the first men to have achieved supreme realisation as a result of the kindling of the inner divine fire, after which he was in a position to show the path to mankind. Hence the many references to his bringing fire to men:

> To Mātariśvan first thou Agni was disclosed, and to Vivasvat through thy noble inward power.[44]

This suspicion is confirmed in the following verse:

> Soon as he sprang to birth that Agni was shown
> forth to Mātariśvan in the highest firmament.[45]

This reference to the 'highest firmament' (*parama-vyoman*) reminds us of St. Paul's hint of being taken up into the third heaven, in other words of having reached a high degree of divine consciousness, a reading which may very well apply to this particular verse of the *Ṛgveda* in so far as Mātariśvan as a human being is concerned. Having reached this

[42] Aurobindo Ghose, *Isha Upanishad*, 2nd rev. ed. (Calcutta, 1924), p. 4.
[43] Ṛgv. III.29.11.
[44] Ṛgv. I.31.3.
[45] Ṛgv. I.143.2.

depth of contemplation, man then understands the meaning of the fire working through all substances and all beings and making all things one by its mere presence. The same fire burns in all.

> Him Mātariśvan brought to us from far away produced by friction from the gods.[46]

Friction is not merely physical, for friction is exertion and therefore occurs at all levels, emotional, intellectual, spiritual as well as physical. It implies resistance and the latter means interaction, effort, conquest, achievement. The gift of the divine spark was originally from the gods, but it had to be kindled and tended by the human being. Further details are given:

> What Mātariśvan piercing formed by friction, herald of all the gods in varied figure is he whom they have set mid human houses.[47]

Neither Sāyaṇa, nor Wilson, nor Griffith observed the fundamentally spiritual significance of this verse. Ideas, especially those expressed in ancient scriptures, can indeed be interpreted at different levels. But one of the greatest symbols of the Vedas, fire, cannot be reduced merely to sex, as was done by the early European symbolists. P. Decharme following an explanation concerning the production of fire in the *Ṛgveda* writes: 'The production of fire was thus compared by the Aryans to an act of generation of which the pramantha was the male instrument, the arani the female instrument.'[48] This is explaining the fire at the lowest level, but that fire which is also the *kavikratu*, the immortal boon to which man aspires, is far more. Decharme does admit 'the ancient assimilation of the human soul to a celestial spark',[49] but soars no higher in his explanation of the production of fire by attrition.

The word translated as 'piercing' (*viṣṭa*) may bear a more spiritual connotation. Mātariśvan by his mental and divine exertion 'pierced'

[46] Ṛgv. III.9.5.
[47] Ṛgv. I.148.1.
[48] P. Decharme, *Mythologie de la Grèce antique* (Paris, 1879), p. 252. The translation is ours.
[49] op. cit., p. 252.

through the ordinary human consciousness penetrating into a level of awareness superior to all empirical inner states, hence termed divine. In other words, he succeeded in kindling the inner fire, the spark latent in every man and biding its time until the 'chalice', which according to the legend the Ṛbhus made fourfold, should be ready. He thus found the path to immortality and exhorted others thereto. He gave of his own fire to men. The friction here refers to the constant pressure exerted by the spiritual essence upon the personality with its incessant falls, failures, reticences, its unwillingness to be relegated to a secondary rank. This is friction indeed. There may also be a play upon the idea with regard to the production of physical fire by friction, but to explain the verse as merely 'the wind penetrating [amidst the fuel] has excited [Agni]', as Wilson following Sāyaṇa has done, is to completely ignore the fundamental meaning of Agni and the role he played throughout antiquity, not only among the Vedic people, but also the Iranians and all other Indo-Europeans.

A very similar verse occurs in *Ṛgveda* VI.16.13, where this time Atharvan, another of the earliest men to have achieved spiritual realisation, is shown as drawing Agni by friction: 'Agni, Atharvan drew thee forth from the lotus flower by rubbing.' This recalls a somewhat similar parallel in a poem of Guñjarīpāda, one verse of which is quoted in M. Eliade's work on Yoga: 'The lotus and the thunder meet together in the middle and through their union Caṇḍālī is ablaze; that blazing fire is in contact with the house of the Ḍombī . . .'[50] The Ṛgvedic verse, like that of Guñjarīpāda, does not stand a literal interpretation; both use highly symbolic language. Thus A. C. Das shows complete lack of insight in his far-fetched attempts at explanations: 'How did Atharvan draw Agni forth from the lotus flower passes our comprehension, unless we suppose that the sparks emitted by striking two flint-stones together were caught by the dry lotus-petals which were thus ignited.'[51] Griffith has a more sensible footnote: '. . . the lotus-flower: apparently a figurative expression for heaven'. Commenting on this note, A. C. Das wonders: '. . . how could Atharvan bring forth Agni from heaven by rubbing?'[52] This is the kind of useless speculation one is led to if one misses the highly symbolic meaning of many Ṛgvedic verses. The lotus flower is one of the most

[50] M. Eliade, *Yoga: Immortality and Freedom*, p. 246.
[51] A. C. Das, *Ṛgvedic Culture* (Calcutta, 1925), p. 74.
[52] op. cit., p. 74.

ancient symbols closely connected with water or the manifested world. In paintings it is depicted as growing out of Viṣṇu's navel whilst he rests upon the waters of space and the serpent of infinity. It images the coming into objective manifestation of all created things and thus symbolises nature. The seeds of the plant are said to contain the miniature shape of what the flower will be when fully grown. The birth of every great soul, such as Osiris, Horus, Gautama, Christ, has always been associated with this flower, whether under the shape of the Oriental lotus or the Occidental lily. The lotus, furthermore, grows from the slime or water to bloom forth into the sunlight, a perfect imagery from which the human mind could read its own history: from the tomb of the body, the soul flowers forth, and only from and through that full flowering can the divine flame, or that jewel in the lotus, be made manifest. There may also be a technical meaning in this drawing of the fire from the lotus by Atharvan. For each of the *cakras* or plexuses or centres in the human constitution has been described as a lotus in the later literature. The heart itself is a lotus. We may wonder whether this was already known in Vedic times. The use of the word *puṣkara* and the root *manth* with reference to Agni seem to be pointers to such a possible knowledge.

The very path that Atharvan followed is expressed as a highly ethical way of life, the only way that can lead to the kindling of the inner fire: 'Atharvan first by sacrifices laid the paths; then, guardian of the law sprang up the loving sun.'[53] The translator, Griffith, here closely follows the Sanskrit original, the meaning of the last part of which is not very clear. 'Having found the divine fire, Atharvan became as the sun to others', is a possible interpretation. Physical fire has no connection with law, sacrifice, or ethics. And so the seer declares: 'They who understand stir thee to action with their thoughts.'[54]

A short allegory on the inner significance of Agni is outlined in *Ṛgveda* IV.1.11–18, in Vāmadeva's highly symbolic language. This is of the greatest interest, as *maṇḍala* IV is considered the oldest of the ten books which make up the collection of hymns, because it shows that in far back times the age-old myth of the finding of the divine flame was already fully expressed in men's minds. Agni, who is enjoined in the tenth verse 'to conduct us—for he knows the way—to all that he enjoys of god-sent riches', first rises in the 'birth-place of holy order',

[53] Ṛgv. I.83.5.
[54] Ṛgv. VIII.44.19.

in the 'bull's lair', the latter being Griffith's rendering of *vṛṣabhasya nīḷe* (Ṛgv. IV.1.12)—two descriptive epithets of utmost importance; the second one, referring not to 'the fuel in which he grows strong', as Griffith so unpoetically explains in a footnote, nor, with all due respect to Sāyaṇa, to 'the nest of the raincloud', but—knowing that the epithet 'bull' is again and again applied to gods, Agni, Indra, Viṣṇu—rather to the abode of the gods, heaven. This reading is confirmed by the first epithet, 'the home of holy order' (*ṛtasya yoni*) which is not merely 'the place of law-appointed sacrifice', in the sense of human ritualistic offering, as Griffith notes, but the foundation of all, the cosmic order (*ṛta*) whence the divine statutes which even the gods must obey. It should be observed that *vṛṣabha* also means 'mighty, powerful', so that a far better translation, and one more in the spirit of the seer's vision, would be 'in the abode of the mighty one'. The next verse (Ṛgv. IV.1.13) shows 'our human fathers', the *ṛṣis*' ancestors, taking their place in that abode: 'Here did our human fathers take their places, fain to fulfil the sacred law of worship.' Thence they drove 'Dawn's teeming milch-kine hid in the mountain-stable, in the cavern'. Two words here claim particular attention, *aśmavraja* and *vavra*, both emphasising the idea of a dark hidden place—the cattle is hidden not merely in the dark cave, but in a rocky mountain cavern. This idea recurs many times in the *Ṛgveda* under different names: *kha* (IV.11.2, where Agni is asked to disclose to the poet his thought, *manīṣa*, hidden as in a well), *guhā nisīdan* (I.67.2) or again *guhā* (I.65.1). The fathers reach out to the hiding place set in the rock; this mountain of spiritual perception, each seer has to climb before he may attain to the inmost of the inmost, the cavern, thence to release the divine rays of light, here the milch-kine imprisoned in the mountain cave or stable. However odd the metaphor of kine for rays may strike the modern mind, it is a recognised symbol, the word *go* used in the plural meaning rays of light. The Vedic civilisation was mainly pastoral, hence the use of bucolic terms. The next two verses continue in like manner showing how the fathers rent the mountain freeing the cattle 'with thought intent upon the booty', as Griffith unfortunately translates *gavyatā manasā*. The word *gavyat* does mean 'desirous of cattle' or of battle or 'ardently desiring'. There is obviously a play upon the word *go* which outwardly follows the bucolic imagery, but the meaning remains that the fathers are intent on, or ardently desiring to find, the rays of light. The fourteenth stanza emphasises the exhilaration of the whole deed:

'Splendid were they when they had rent the mountain.' The intensive form *marmṛjata* from ($\sqrt{\ }$*mṛj*, 'to purify') would certainly strike a most incongruous note if physical booty was meant. 'They sang their song prepared to free the cattle.' 'They found the light (*vidanta jyotiḥ*), 'with holy hymns they worshipped' (*cakṛpanta dhībhiḥ*). Statements like these are clear hints that the poet is speaking in metaphors. However, the latter translation is wholly insufficient. *Cakṛpanta* ($\sqrt{\ }$*kṛp*, 'to lament') has the connotation of chanting (or = $\sqrt{\ }$*kḷp* 'to fashion'). *Dhībhiḥ*, from *dhī*, means visionary thought, an actual perception at a higher level of cognition. Aurobindo elucidates: '. . . *dhī* is the thought-power, intellect or understanding. It is intermediate between the normal mentality represented by the combination of Indra and Vāyu and the *Ṛtam* or Truth-consciousness.'[55] This verse is a characteristic example of the Vedic belief that by means of certain sacred incantations which in themselves were prayers for worship, the devotee could break through to non-physical levels of existence. The *ṛṣi* uses the hymn as a vehicle (*ratha*), it is stated many times: 'For Jātavedas [*i.e.* Agni] worthy of our praise will we frame this eulogy as 'twere a car.'[56] Agni himself is considered the charioteer, the thought which expresses itself as the chant being the car.[57]

The fathers broke through the confining walls of the ordinary consciousness, freeing thereby the rays of the divine awareness which, one may conclude, then penetrated to the empirical level: 'Then afterwards, they looked around, awakened, when first they held that heaven-allotted treasure.'[58] This verse is most significant and particularly so the verb 'awakened' (*bubudhānā*) which strikes the keynote of an awakening to the heaven-allotted treasure. After they have become alive to these new realities, the fathers (*pitṛs*) exclaim: 'All gods are in all houses.'[59] This surely means that the divine or *ātman*, the jewel hidden away, dwells in the human, the godly powers visioned by the *ṛṣis* as actual entities have their counterpart in the human being. 'Let the truth be to the thought,' or understanding or vision, as we should translate the end of the Ṛgvedic verse IV.1.18. In other words, let truth take shape and fulfil-

[55] Aurobindo, *On the Veda*, p. 79.
[56] Ṛgv. I.94.1.
[57] *Vide* Ṛgv. IV.10.2: 'For thou hast ever been the car-driver, of noble strength, lofty sacrifice and rightful judgement.'
[58] Ṛgv. IV.1.18.
[59] Ṛgv. IV.1.18: *viśve viśvāsu duryāsu devā.*

ment in the vision, the vision is truth. The whole poem is a perfect allegory of spiritual birth brought about through the agency of Agni.

The very same idea is expressed in another hymn giving a similar story, where the rock (*adri*) which the fathers must burst open is again stressed: 'Our sires with lauds burst e'en the firm-set fortress, yea, the Aṅgiras, with roar, the mountain.'[60] By their praises, by their clamour (*rava*), 'they made for us a way to reach high heaven', 'they found us day, light', and so on. Obviously, these early people strove after the undecaying light which mankind has ever associated with heaven, and not after booty in the guise of cattle hidden in rocks.[61]

Agni's 'own home' (*sva dama*)[62] calls for a deeper consideration. It is the 'birth-place of harmony' (*ṛtasya yoni*), the 'abode of the mighty one' (*vṛṣabhasya nīḷa*),[63] that home in which he is enjoined 'to shine forth . . . as guardian of the law' (Ṛgv. III.10.2), that is, the divine cosmic order which is the truth, for he is 'born in holy order' (Ṛgv. VI.7.1), thus confirming that the 'bull's lair', to follow Griffith's translation, is indeed the bucolic symbol of the seat of celestial harmony. The very first hymn of the Ṛgvedic collection strikes the keynote of all the *maṇḍalas*. For everything that Agni represents to his worshippers, the very essence of Vedic thought, is there expressed in a most skilful way. Agni is invoked as the 'divine ministrant of sacrifice' (Ṛgv. I.1.1.) placed before ought else, the 'treasure bestower' of 'wise insight' (*kavikratu*), of 'most glorious inspiration' (Ṛgv. I.1.6). He 'thrives' in his 'own sphere' (Ṛgv. I.1.8), that of *ṛta* or the truth, because he is the 'shepherd of holy order' (*gopaṃ ṛtasya*). Thus whatever good he will do for the worshipper is his 'truth' (*satya*), that truth or treasure (*ratna*) which he always bestows, and which in later times was called by the Buddhist monks the 'present of the *dharma*', considered the supreme gift.

To interpret the sense of Agni's growing in his sphere as merely 'the sacrificial hall . . . in which the fire (*agni*) increases as the oblations of clarified butter are poured upon it', as Griffith assumes,[64] or to explain it, as Macdonell does, as merely the 'receptacle on the altar'

[60] Ṛgv. I.71.

[61] *Cf.* the rock struck by Moses from which the refreshing water spurted out. Old Testament, Exodus XVII.6; Numbers XX.10, 11 etc. *Cf.* also Ṛgv. I.93.4: 'Ye found the light, the single light for many.'

[62] Ṛgv. I.75.5.

[63] *Vide* Ṛgv. IV.1.12.

[64] R. T. H. Griffith, *The Hymns of the Ṛigveda* (Benares, 1896), vol. I, p. 2.

in which 'the sacrificial fire . . . flames up'[65] is to reduce the grand conception of *ṛta* to the puny dimensions of a physical man-made altar. *Ṛta* implies that perfect harmony existing between the essence of being (*sat*) and its activity: the spontaneous rightness observable in the majestic movement of the stars, the recurrence of the seasons, the unswerving alternance of day and night, the unerring rhythm of birth, growth, death, the universal equilibrium, the rhythm which is the very breath of divine action. All cosmic processes are rooted in *ṛta*, are effects or reflections of an inner harmony, a divine order, a supreme law, expressed in the vedic word *ṛta*.

The sacrifice of which Agni is the supreme ministrant is one aspect of the cosmic truth: at the level of the ritual it aims at reflecting the divine sacrifice on which the world is founded,[66] at the personal level at mirroring the universal action: by means of his self-sacrifice, of which the outer rite is but the symbol, man allows the divine powers to grow within himself and accomplish their work of purification and harmony. Hence the emphasis upon the path of sacrifice trod by all the holy men mentioned in the *Ṛgveda*: Manu, Ṛbhu, Atharvan, Aṅgiras, Mātariśvan and others. From the human standpoint, the microcosmic view, this is the supreme meaning of Agni the sacrificial priest, the envoy (*dūta*) who ranges between heaven and earth, the fire which links man to god, the choice-worthy 'guest', immortal among mortals, a significance Western exegesis has hardly touched upon. Thus the many statements as to Agni's fuel can be understood in a much deeper sense than the mere obvious physical one. 'When mortal man presents to thee, immortal god, Agni, his fuel, or his sacrificial gift, then thou art his . . . messenger.'[67] And: 'Man's sacrificial food hath sharpened like an axe, for brightness, him the sage of men, the people's lord.'[68] These are verses which call for more than a cursory thought, or a literal rendering. So Śrī Aurobindo comments:

> We must remember that the oblation (*havya*) signifies always action (*karma*) and each action of mind or body is regarded as a giving of our plenty into the cosmic being and the cosmic intention. Agni, the divine Will, is that which stands behind the human will in its

[65] A. A. Macdonell, *Vedic Reader* (London, Oxford University Press, 1960), p. 9.
[66] *Vide* Ṛgv. X.90 and X.130.
[67] Ṛgv. X.91.11.
[68] Ṛgv. III.2.10.

works . . . But it is in proportion as we learn to subjugate the ego and compel it to bow down in every act to the universal Being and to serve consciously in its least movements the supreme Will, that Agni himself takes form in us. The Divine Will becomes present and conscient in a human mind and enlightens it with the Divine Knowledge. Thus it is that man can be said to form by his toil the great Gods.[69]

J. Gonda shows in his translation of *Ṛgveda* X.114.6 as '. . . the sages, having produced, by means of higher wisdom, the sacrifice' his understanding of the close connection between the sacrifice (*yajña*) and that wise apprehension of truth which can only occur at a level out of all relation to the ordinary consciousness.[70] The Vedic sacrifice is a far loftier conception than has hitherto been supposed. It is a universal process to which all things from atoms to human beings are subjected—the eternal give and take: at the lowest level a preying, as it seems to the mind, at the highest an eternal self-gift.[71] Hence the universal application of the following statement: 'This sacrifice, the hub of the world.'[72] The particular Vedic ritual is hereby the symbolic enactment of what constantly occurs in the cosmos. Of this grand cosmic conception, Agni is the divine ministrant. 'All men . . . truly share thy Godhead, while they keep, in their accustomed ways, eternal law.'[73] Man thus partakes of the eternal sacrifice through Agni, the immortal guest in mortal houses, 'the household friend who knows all things that be' who 'drives the chariot of the lofty ordinance, Agni most active', 'the great high priest of the gods'.[74]

The term *vaiśvānara*, Agni's distinguishing epithet, itself points to the omnipresence of Agni in man. Derived from the root *viś* ('to settle in, enter') and *nṛ* ('man'), it means that which is present or residing in all men, or as a verse states, that which is found at 'the centre of the people, sustaining men like a deep-founded pillar' (Ṛgv. I.59.1). It is the inmost fire of each human being, that fire which 'supports'

[69] Aurobindo, *On the Veda*, pp. 294–5.
[70] *Vide* J. Gonda, *The Vision of the Vedic Poets*, p.53.
[71] *Cf.* Revelation XIII.8: 'The lamb immolated from the foundation of the world . . .'
[72] Ṛgv. I.164.35.
[73] Ṛgv. I.68.2.
[74] *Vide* Ṛgv. III.2.8.

the body and mind, as it does the whole universe. So when the seers declared that 'in choosing Agni, men choose one who has the wisdom of a seer',[75] their statement certainly is much more profound than appears at first sight. Seership, wisdom, the highest characteristics to which man is heir, the gifts of the *ātman* or Self, are here unhesitatingly identified with Agni. Śrī Aurobindo's description may now cease to appear unfounded or exaggerated: 'His is a flame of force instinct with the light of divine knowledge. Agni is the seer-will in the universe, unerring in all its works . . . the immortal worker in man.'[76]

The specific mentions of Mātariśvan's bringing fire to certain men of ancient India (*e.g.* the Bhṛgus)[77] give occasion for some of the most extraordinary and elusive of Ṛgvedic myths. Among these are the legend of the Ṛbhus, the three brothers, sons of Sudhanvan, called grandsons or great grandsons of Manu, the first mortal, thus showing that they are human beings who gained their immortality through their own exertion.

Successive steps can be detected in the handing on of the mystery of the fire. First, the 'deities produced thee, a god, to be a light unto the *ārya*'[78]— unto the noble-minded one or him who is spiritually ready; these noble souls 'engendered Agni in heaven';[79] then, such exalted human beings as Mātariśvan and Atharvan, by their spiritual exertion, discovered him and brought him to men. 'As 'twere some goodly treasure Mātariśvan brought, as a gift, the glorious priest [Agni] to Bhṛgu.'[80] Then, 'the Bhṛgus stablished thee among mankind for men like a treasure, beauteous, easy to invoke; thee Agni as a herald and choice worthy guest, as an auspicious friend to the celestial race'.[81] The divine fire was passed on to the Ṛbhus who 'skillfully urged the work' which 'won them everlasting life, serving with holy rites,

[75] Ṛgv. V.11.4.
[76] Aurobindo, *On the Veda*, pp. 400–1.
[77] According to Max Müller, the Bhṛgus were a tribe who were accepted by the Brāhmaṇic community, but had no Vedic gods. They are considered an ancient priestly family among the first Aryans who entered India. The Ṛbhus were ascribed to them as gods. In later times there seems to have been some confusion as to both names.
[78] Ṛgv. I.59.2.
[79] Ṛgv. X.88.10.
[80] Ṛgv. I.60.1.
[81] Ṛgv. I.58.6.

pious with noble acts'.[82] The emphasis on holiness is again significant. The Ṛbhus in turn 'served him in the home of waters, set him of old in houses of the living'[83]—a most suggestive stanza of which another parallel will be quoted later.

By means of a juxtaposition of pertinent verses there is apparent an archaic *paraṃparā*—the handing down from generation to generation of the secret or supreme knowledge, the finding of the flame divine which to the Vedic people was *ātma-vidyā*, Self-realisation, the heart of their religion. The *ṛṣis*, those 'children of the gods',[84] call upon Agni 'as erst did Bhṛgus, Manus, Aṅgiras',[85] as 'Aurva Bhṛgu used, as Apnavāna used'[86] to call, Aurva being said to be the grandson of Bhṛgu. Again, Apnavāna of the family of Bhṛgu as well as the 'Bhṛgus caused Agni to shine bright-coloured in the wood, spreading from home to home'.[87] This verse may, like 'Now all gods abide in all houses' (Ṛgv. IV.1.18), be taken literally. Yet in the light of the above commentaries and those which are to follow there are reasons for believing in a double meaning in these expressions. Physical fire cannot 'win everlasting life' (Ṛgv. III.60.3); it is also not endowed with 'deepest knowledge' (Ṛgv. I.71.10) and does not remove hatred, want and sorrow.[88] A curious verse occurs in *Ṛgveda* X.46.7: 'His are the fires, eternal, purifying, that make the houses move, whose smoke is shining.' To this Griffith comments: 'This seems to be what the words *damām aritrā* should mean though how flames can be thus qualified is not clear.'[89] Only the inner fire of the spirit can make the human being progress along the path. This again is a perfect example of Vedic imagery.

In the few hymns addressed to them, the Ṛbhus are enjoined to help man find the path to eternal life as they did themselves. The symbols used to express their particular labours are one of the great keys to Vedic symbolism.[90] The Ṛbhus' feats are summed up in *Ṛgveda* IV.35

[82] *Vide* Ṛgv. III.60.3.
[83] Ṛgv. II.4.2.
[84] Ṛgv. X.62.4.
[85] Ṛgv. VIII.43.13.
[86] Ṛgv. VIII.91.4.
[87] Ṛgv. IV.7.1.
[88] *Vide* Ṛgv IV.11.5,6.
[89] R. T. H. Griffith, *The Hymns of the Ṛigveda*, vol. II, p. 447.
[90] Max Müller found a close connection between *ṛbhu* and Orpheus and the myths woven around these two names. *Vide* also F. Nève, *Essai sur le mythe des Ribhavas* (Paris, 1847).

and 36 in the colourful language typical of the seer Vāmadeva, but are referred to in many another hymn. As Aurobindo points out: 'The Ṛbhus are artisans of immortality.'[91] This quality is well brought out in the following stanza: 'Ye whom your artist skill hath raised to godhead.'[92] They fashion car, cow, chalice and so on for a specific purpose and through, or by means of, inspiration or visionary insight, out of their own mind.[93] Because of 'the mighty powers wherewith ye formed the chalices', because of 'the thought by which ye drew the cow from out the hide', 'the intellect wherewith ye wrought the two bay steeds', the Ṛbhus became immortal.[94] The suggestion that the Ṛbhus achieved this particular labour by the 'power of speech' (*śacī*) is similar to the *ṛṣis'* idea of the objective effect of the power of incantation (*mantra*).

The words of power referred to again in *Ṛgveda* I.161.9 should be examined, as they might throw at least some light on the whole question of the Ṛbhus' deification. The order in which these words are presented is rather remarkable. First, the 'waters' are stated to be excellent. Then, the second Ṛbhu claims: 'Most excellent is Agni.' The power which Agni personifies recurs in the third 'word': 'Another praised to many a one the lightning cloud.' This refers to the lightning aspect of Agni in its highest spiritual sense, the destructive or regenerating flame divine. The word 'lightning cloud' (*vadharyantī*) brings to mind Indra's famous weapon, the 'thunderbolt' (*vajra*), about which J. Gonda explains: '. . . the "thunderbolt weapon" . . . is applied to various objects or entities which are instrumental in producing what is good and useful for man . . . Being a manifestation of celestial light it could, then, have been credited also with a role in the process of the manifestation of "visions".'[95] We have here a clue as to the significance of Agni in his lightning form closely connected with Indra, the wielder of the thunderbolt. Agni, in this specific aspect, is that flash of instant all-illuminating vision which suddenly rends man's mental sky, and Indra, the personification of the mind which through concentration helps to bring about the required onepointedness. Many of the legends referring to the latter as rending the mountain and releasing the cows have this psychological background, apart from any other references.

[91] Aurobindo, *On the Veda*, p. 352.
[92] Ṛgv. IV.35.8.
[93] *Vide* Ṛgv. IV.36.2.
[94] *Vide* Ṛgv. III.60.2.
[95] J. Gonda, *The Vision of the Vedic Poets*, p. 85.

In the second verse of the Ṛgvedic hymn I.161, Agni is made to speak and to command the making of the chalice (*camasa*) into four parts. The Ṛbhus then 'shaped the cups, speaking the words of truth' (verse 9). Following Aurobindo's clue, we can assume that these four cups, the fourfold chalice, are the ancient Vedic poetised way of expressing the consciousness of man which must be perfected upon the four planes of its activity—physical, psychic (including the emotional), intellectual and spiritual. The role Agni plays in this process of progressive perfection is made perfectly clear in the following verse:

> For glory Agni, day by day, thou liftest up
> the mortal man to highest immortality (*amṛtatva*).[96]

Thus closely allied with this gift of fire which early perfected men brought to their descendants is that of immortality, hence the bond between Agni, the flame, and Soma, the nectar of bliss, both of whom are sometimes considered as the two poles of the one essence. Agni is described as the 'guardian of Soma' (Ṛgv. X.45.5). Similarly, Soma is styled the 'guardian of holy order', Agni's birth-home in *Ṛgveda* IX.73.8. This association alone ought to point out that the myth of Mātariśvan's gift of fire to mankind has far deeper connotations than are usually admitted. Both Agni and Soma, born in 'heaven' (*dyu*) or on the 'mountain' (*adri*), are characteristically manifested on earth by the pressure either of wooden sticks or of stones—a pressure, friction or rubbing which, as shown, has also a figurative sense. Both when manifested in the human being may have the same effect, that of exhilaration: 'Like kindled fire, inflame me . . . illumine us!'[97] Thus is the song of the poet invoking Soma. Both are brought together and differentiated in this one statement: 'Mātariśvan fetched one of you from heaven. The falcon rent the other from the mountain rock.'[98] Mātariśvan, as the lightning or cosmic aspect of Agni on the one hand, or, on the other hand, as that aspect manifested in a perfected human, fetched the flame from heaven and brought it to Indra who represents the mind in Vedic symbology. But the falcon, or eagle (*śyena*), is also that same flame, for elsewhere it is identified with Agni, 'falcon of the firmament' (Ṛgv. VII.15.4); here it wrenches or churns up (*mantha*) the draught of

[96] Ṛgv. I.31.7.
[97] Ṛgv. VIII.48.6.
[98] Ṛgv. I.93.6.

immortality from the very rock (of matter). The mountain rock may bear various meanings as for example those inaccessible heights where spiritual realisation takes place. Soma is 'taken from yon loftiest heaven' (Ṛgv. IV.26.6), as well as from the rock. Here (Ṛgv. I.93.6), interpreting *adri* as 'matter', there would then be the age-old idea that through the tomb of the body (or rock of matter) man rises to the glory of the perfect soul (*siddha*), or becomes immortal.

Another expression of this celebrated legend, perpetuated for Europe in the Greek Prometheus, appears in *Ṛgveda* IV.26 and 27. Here the falcon 'confined by one hundred fortresses'[99] yet flies forth to heaven to snatch from its keeper the nectar of immortality which he then offers to Indra. The Brāhmaṇas refer to this legend in various ways, changing Agni or the falcon into the *gāyatrī*. The meaning remains the same—a poetic or mythical account of the flame spirit metaphorically descending from its own sphere, where it has quaffed the beverage of immortal bliss, to make its mortal host man, or mind, the god of the senses, personified in Indra, partake of its nature. This interpretation can be compared with M. Bloomfield's painstaking proof that '. . . the entire legend resolves itself into the description of one of the most simple and salient natural phenomena. . . . When the summer-storm breaks out, the lightning, the eagle, breaks from the cloud, and with it comes the rush of the heavenly fluid upon the earth'.[100] One may wonder how the meteorological phenomenon of the lightning can bestow on the mortal supreme immortality, for Soma is Agni's gift. It is through Agni's 'mental powers' (*kratu*) that the gods 'were made immortal' (Ṛgv. VI.7.4).

Agni's lightning aspect has far deeper implications than has hitherto been suspected. Of the many riddles scattered through the *Ṛgveda* there are perhaps none more tantalising than those connected with this cosmic side. Several perfect hieroglyphics could be noted. One such appears in *Ṛgveda* II.35.9, where the 'son of waters' (*apāṃ napāt*), one expression of Agni, is said to rise 'upright' amidst the waters, the 'prone', that nurse him: 'The Son of waters has occupied the lap of the prone, [himself] upright, clothing himself in lightning.'[101] Here is

[99] Ṛgv. IV.27.1.
[100] M. Bloomfield, 'Contributions to the Interpretation of the Veda. 1. The Legend of Soma and the Eagle', *Journal of the American Oriental Society*, vol. XVI (1896), pp. 23–4.
[101] Macdonell's translation.

painted the spirit-flame descending as the lightning into the 'waters', the 'deep' or chaos of Genesis; the vertical line of dynamic life forming with the horizontal line of all-inclusive substance the cross of generation, that cross used as a symbol of manifestation long before the Christians adopted it. A similar hieroglyphic confirms the above meaning:

> Deep in the ocean lies the bolt with waters compassed round about,
> and in continuous onward flow the floods their tribute bring to it.[102]

The picture here takes a step further: it shows the bolt or flame immersed in mundane existence (*saṃsāra*) yet remaining the king to whom all created things—the floods—pay homage.

In connection with this aspect of divinity embedded in the veils or billows of matter, there are other riddles which throw further light on the meaning of the fire, or bird of heaven coming down to earth and flying back whence he came:

> Dark the descent: the birds are golden-coloured; up to the heaven they fly robed in the waters. Again they descend from the seat of order, and all the earth is moistened with their fatness.[103]

The 'bird' has ever symbolised the divine spirit. The colour that describes these birds—for the text uses the plural (*harayaḥ suparṇāḥ*)—should be noted. These descend into the dark realms of matter (*kṛṣṇaṃ niyānam*, literally 'black the entry') where they gather experience, thence re-ascend to heaven whence they came, now 'robed in the waters', the implication of this description being that matter is by the impact of spirit enriched, lifted up or spiritualised. The word *ghṛta*, so very poorly translated as 'fatness' by Griffith, is the illuminating *seed* of the flame. 'Butter indeed means seed', says the *Śatapatha-Brāhmaṇa* (I.9.2.7). For Griffith, the whole verse refers to the meteorological phenomenon of rain. Such an interpretation takes no account of the fundamental meaning of bird (*suparṇa*), waters (*ap*), the seat of order (*ṛta*), heaven (*dyu*) and seed (*ghṛta*). Furthermore, there is a hint as to the coming back to earth of the pilgrim birds (*ta ā-avavṛtrant-sadanād ṛtasya*), a definite turning back from the seat of order, in other words, to the doctrine of *punar-janma*, the return to incarnation, a doctrine

102 Ṛgv. VIII.89.9 (VIII.100.9 according to Max Müller's numbering).
103 Ṛgv. I.164.47.

which is implied in some verses of the same hymn, particularly in Ṛgv. I.164.31.

The secret of discovering Agni, a secret obviously mastered by the ancient *ṛṣis*, is hinted at in one of the most significant verses of the *Ṛgveda*:

> He, bearing in his hand all manly might, crouched in the cavern, struck the gods with fear. Men, filled with understanding, find him there, when they have sung prayers (*mantras*) formed within their heart.[104]

The words 'crouched in the cavern', 'filled with understanding' not merely anticipate the 'cave of the heart' where resides the *ātman* of the Upaniṣads, but clearly indicate that the seers had knowledge of the existence of the divine spark in man, that it dwells in the inmost core of the human being and that it can be aroused by means of prayer and meditation.

This secret place is the repository of wealth as was to be made plain in the Upaniṣads. 'He who knows this [space within the heart] attains eternal and all-sufficient treasures.'[105] Men, claims the Vedic *ṛṣi*, 'loving the loving one' (Ṛgv. I.71.1), can but prosper and reap 'riches' (*rayi*). This latter word occurs so often in prayers addressed to Agni that the kind of 'wealth' which the fire bestows upon the worshipper ought to be examined. For Agni is the 'treasure-lord of treasures' (*rayi patī rayiṇām*, Ṛgv. I.72.1) through whom 'one obtains wealth' (Ṛgv. I.1.3). What is this 'highest treasure' (*varṣiṣṭha-ratna*) which he 'gained by his own nature' (Ṛgv. III.26.8), which enabled him to look abroad over heaven and earth? In the same order of thought Indra is begged in *Ṛgveda* VIII.13.5 to 'bring us wealth manifold which finds the light of heaven'. These verses, as so many others, hold the clue as to their fundamental meaning. He who cherishes 'right judgment' (Ṛgv. IV.10.1)—who is 'pure mental power', as Griffith translates *kratu*—'holds all knowledge in his grasp even as the felly rounds the wheel' (Ṛgv. II.5.3). The meaning of *kavya* given as 'endowed with the qualities of a sage' (Monier-Williams) points to a far deeper significance than comes out in the translation: Agni is inspired with wisdom of the highest order such as can still be met among the *ṛṣis* of modern India,

[104] Ṛgv. I.67.2.
[105] *Chāndogya-Upaniṣad* III.12.8.

that consciousness of the Supreme, a consciousness fully expressed by Ramana Maharshi or Aurobindo. Similarly, the word *kratu*, as Aurobindo points out, connotes 'power effective of action', will. These are Agni's 'highest treasure'. He is 'passing wise', 'a seer'[106] with the seer's wisdom, the 'finder of the light' whom men revere in their heart (Ṛgv. III.26.1), and that which brings utmost union among men (Ṛgv. X.191.1).

It is thus not surprising that in the seer's ecstasy Agni, 'though holding many gifts for men', yet seems to 'humble the higher powers of each wise ordainer' (Ṛgv. I.72.1). Hence, the treasures of him whose 'ecstasy is most mighty, whose mental power is most splendid' (Ṛgv. I.127.9), the riches implored are the grace of divine illumination. The plea 'chasing with light our sin away, O Agni, shine thou wealth on us' (Ṛgv. I.97.1) points to the quality of the wealth demanded. He is implored to 'urge us to strength and holy thought' (Ṛgv. I.27.11), as Griffith translates, or '. . . to stimulate the seer or poet . . . into an effort to obtain a "vision" and vāja', as J. Gonda explains.[107] His is the power of visionary insight, for 'he, the ocean, the foundation of riches, of many births, shines forth from our heart' (Ṛgv. X.5.1).

Thus when it is said that 'men have kindled Agni in the threefold abode' (Ṛgv. V.11.2), the meaning should now be far more significant than the mere outward gesture of the ritual kindling. It is clearly stated that Agni is not fully expressed on earth: 'He is kept secret though his flames are bright.'[108] Another verse asks: 'When may that principle of thy godhood (*devasya cetanam*) be made unceasingly manifest?'[109] The rite of kindling the fire symbolises the inner setting ablaze which occurs at the three levels of the human being; the blending of the three fires within man—of matter, mind and spirit—a blending which heralds the delivered soul. Agni is man's home in the very depths of his being, the dynamic might at the heart of men, gods and cosmos, the very cause of their coming into active existence, of their developing and, in the case of the first two, of their partaking of immortality. He is thus the manifested expression of 'that One who breathed breathless-ly by itself' (Ṛgv. X.129.2), the 'seer-will' (Aurobindo's translation of *kavi-kratu*). All things are the 'robes' Agni assumes. In the *Kaṭha-*

[106] *Vide* Ṛgv. VI.14.2.
[107] J. Gonda, *The Vision of the Vedic Poets*, p. 98.
[108] Ṛgv. IV.7.6.
[109] Ṛgv. IV.7.2.

Upaniṣad he is identified with the Supreme: 'This verily is That.'[110] So also in the *Bhagavad-Gītā*: 'I having become the fire of life. . . .'[111] Deity is equated with fire, the pulse which gives breath to all.

But Agni can be found only by the pure and the strong:

> They who are free from death, fain for him purified three splendours of the mighty Agni, circling all. To man for his enjoyment, one of these they gave; the other two have passed into the sister sphere.[112]

The word *bhuja*, here translated 'enjoyment', also means 'welfare, weal'. For man's own salvation, one of the splendours or kindlings of Agni was given to mankind. The other two are beyond human conception. So the *ātman*[113] to which Agni leads man is the most dynamic of the splendours to which he is heir. But the purifying fire brooks no dross. The ancient sages knew this and allowed no one to be fully initiated into the mysteries of life and death and therefore of the supreme spirit, before he had thoroughly purified himself in thought, word and deed. As the *Atharvaveda* hints:

> Since Agni, we through *tapas*, are kindling the fire of the spirit, may we be dear to the Veda.[114]

Only the pure in mind and body can stand the tremendous impact of the flame divine; otherwise the shattering effect may be deadly or throw the man off his balance for life. Hence the age-old injunctions, found in all religions, as to purification. Each and every impure tendency in thought and action must be laid upon the altar of sacrifice, must become Agni's fuel, before one may hope to find the *ātman* beyond the human personality. Hence the Christian baptism of fire:

> He that cometh after me is mightier than I . . . He shall baptise you

[110] *Kaṭha-Upaniṣad* IV.8: *etad-vai tat.*
[111] *Bhagavad-Gītā* XV.14: *ahaṃ vaiśvānaro bhūtvā.*
[112] Ṛgv. III.2.9.
[113] The Conception of *ātman* as found in later Vedic literature may not have been fully developed in Ṛgvedic times. Nevertheless, the *ṛṣis* had an inkling of something highest in man which we chose to call *ātman* and which to them was the essence of Agni.
[114] Ath.veda VII.61.1. The translation is that of A. C. Bose, *Hymns from the Vedas* (London, 1966), p. 71.

> with the Holy Ghost and with fire . . . He will burn up the chaff with unquenchable fire.[115]

Some Buddhists claim fire destroys the body of an *arahant*, its essence makes him immortal.

There are several references in the *Ṛgveda* to Agni's purifying action. In a hymn of the eighth *maṇḍala* he is called 'far-spreading, purifier, him whose path is black' (Ṛgv. VIII.23.19). Elsewhere he is said to be a 'priest with purifying tongue' (Ṛgv. VI.11.2).

Another striking example is found in a hymn to Soma, where Agni's cleansing, burning action is described. A literal rendering of the verse would run thus:

> Ready is thy filter (*pavitra*) Lord of prayer; supreme, thou pervadest each and every limb. The cold, unripened vessel cannot receive that; only vessels made ready receive that.[116]

The 'filter', metaphorically speaking, refers to the human organism. The words which in the text point to the maturing process for which Agni is responsible, or to its lack, are *śṛta* ('boiled, dressed, ready'), *atapta-tanū* ('unheated body') and *āma* ('raw')—each and every one implying heat or its lack and thus the action of fire. When all the impurities have fallen away, the 'filter' or human organism is ready, the vehicle or personality stands transparent, capable of fully reflecting the inner ruler. The result is succinctly described in the Christian scriptures: Jesus, according to St. Matthew, took three of his disciples on to a high mountain apart, and 'he was transfigured before them and his face did shine as the sun and his raiment was white as the light'.[117] The kindled flame of spirit glowed so powerfully that it manifested even at the physical level and the three disciples who were by his side fell upon their faces, overawed at the divine presence. This is the action of fire.

The conception of 'maturing' also appears in a rather strange hymn, *Ṛgveda* X.16.1, whose main purport is cremation, but where Agni is asked not to 'burn up' the dead man, nor quite consume him. . . . 'When thou hast matured him then send him on his way unto the Fathers.' This verse hints at the belief in the purification of the flame

[115] N.T. Math. III.11. 12.
[116] Ṛgv. IX.83.1.
[117] *Vide* N.T. Math. XVII.1.

not merely at the physical level, but also apparently at the psychological level—since the man is dead—with the idea that only after this process of 'maturing' is over can the dead man join the *pitṛs* or the elect.

Closely connected with purification is strength, for only the strong can stand the flame, or the purifying process. 'Agni, the wise, bestows the might of heroes, grants strengthening food, preparing it for nectar.'[118] The words *vīrya* ('vigour, virility') and *vāja* ('might') emphasise the kind of vigorous energy, or heroic soul-power, that Agni grants, for his is the dynamic force, the cosmic will that manifests in man as in the universe and that nothing can impede. Such heroic dynamism prepares (√ *bhūṣ*, 'to strive after, care for') the worshipper for the strong drink the soul covets. Here the idea of 'valour' and 'striving' is plainly brought out. Only those who are ready—purified and brave—can gain the boon of immortality.

The purifying aspect is also the punitive or destructive aspect of Agni which in later times became more and more emphasised. In the *Ṛgveda* many references to this side of Agni's nature may be found, but although they do emphasise the terror at the sight of the devouring flames, there seems to be far more admiration and exhilaration at the beauty displayed than absolute horror or fear at the destruction perpetrated:

> Dread and resistless he destroys the forests.[119]

> He strikes with terror like a dart shot forth . . . to him lead all your ways; may we attain the kindled god as cows their home at eve.[120]

The latter verse plainly shows that in spite of his terrifying effects, Agni remains the flame, the ultimate hearth to which all men are enjoined to reach out. His task is but to 'smite down the sinner like a tree with lightning flash' (Ṛgv. VI.8.5).

Paradoxically, as it may seem, fire is also love, love the dynamo, the magnet, the foundation of the world. In the *Atharvaveda*, Agni is identified with *kāma* ('desire, will, love'),[121] and in the *Ṛgveda*, he is the

[118] Ṛgv. III.25.2.
[119] Ṛgv. VI.6.5.
[120] Ṛgv. I.66.4, 5.
[121] *Vide* Ath.veda IX.2.

personification of the great virtues of friendliness[122] and fatherhood.

> Agni, men seek thee as a father with their prayers, win thee, bright formed, to brotherhood and holy act.[123]

This verse reveals that even in his compassionate aspect, Agni retains his active, masculine essence, remains the essentially dynamic pole of creation, the father, the mover of all things. He is sought as a refuge: 'Be thou a refuge, bright one, to the singer, a shelter, bounteous lord, to those who worship.'[124] He is looked upon as the great intercessor or mediator, the high priest between gods and men who is asked to 'remit entirely our offences' (Ṛgv. IV.12.4), to make us 'sinless' (*anāga*),[125] to 'forgive whatever sin we have committed' (Ṛgv. VII.93.7).

Fire the creator, fire the preserver, fire the destroyer! The roots of the Hindu trinity go far back into the past of Indian religious thought, to the visionary insights of the Vedic *ṛṣis*. Burning in the heart of the sun, of the earth, of man and of all creatures, Agni is the witness to the *ṛṣis*' knowledge of the great forces hidden in nature and in man, and of the fundamental oneness of all things, however manifold the vestures assumed. Through the furthest stars right down to the inmost core of every human being throbs the same dynamic pulse, the fire of creation, the warmth of preservation, the bolt of destruction, Agni, the flame divine. As the *Muṇḍaka-Upaniṣad* recapitulates:

> That which is flaming, subtler than the subtle; on which the worlds are fixed with all their dwellers; that is the imperishable Absolute.[126]

[122] *Vide* Ṛgv. I.44.10; 99.1.
[123] Ṛgv. II.1.9.
[124] Ṛgv. I.58.9. *Cf.* Ṛgv. I.31.10 and IV.11.5, 6.
[125] *Vide* Ṛgv. IV.12.4.
[126] *Muṇḍaka-Up.* II.2.2.

7 *Meister Eckehart —Mystic or Yogin?*

If Yoga and mysticity[1] be taken in their *traditional* forms, the curate of Thuringia and prior of Erfurt, friar Eckehart, was neither the one nor the other. However, as will be seen, elements of both basic phenomena of religious life are contained in his teaching. Yoga and mysticity share one important characteristic; both are forms of expression of the religious or spiritual 'drive', man's need to forge ahead to his original home, the ultimate reality. But while mysticity, in its different modes and degrees, is a primary constituent of all higher religions, Yoga is to be recognised as a specific Indian creation. This does not imply that Yoga does not appear in the cultures of the adjoining countries, but it is generally no longer represented there in its pure form as, for example, the Japanese *dhyāna* or Zen school exemplifies. Anyway, it would be wrong to speak of an Egyptian, a Mohammedan or Hebrew Yoga, as was done by W. J. Flagg.[2]

Mysticity is here understood as that mode of the religious in which the transcendent reality is aspired to by an enstrangement from the phenomenal world and an absorption into the depths of one's own being with the aim of realising the Absolute in its pure nakedness. This qualification of the term mysticity can also, with a greater or lesser degree of accuracy, be applied to Yoga, as can be seen from such traditional definitions as 'Yoga is indifference [towards worldly objects]',[3] 'Yoga is enstasis'[4] and 'Yoga is the connection of the empirical self with the transcendent Self'.[5] The main distinction

[1] We prefer to use this archaic English word in the present discussion in order to clearly distinguish between the genuine mystical teaching and practice (in German *Mystik*) and the misty and mysterious mysticism (in German *Mystizismus*).

[2] W. J. Flagg, *Yoga or Transformation* (New York, London, 1898).

[3] BhG II.48: *samatvaṃ yoga ucyate.*

[4] YBh. I.1: *yogaḥ samādhiḥ.*

[5] *Yoga-Yājñavalkya* I.44: *saṃyogo yoga ity-ukto jīva-ātma-parama-ātmanoḥ.*

between Yoga and mysticity lies in the fact that the former is more experimental and scientific in nature, while the latter—both being taken in their traditional forms—is rather emotional-intuitive-ecstatic.[6] This difference makes itself apparent in the path and method as well as, in some respect, in the final goal.

The Yogic path (*yoga-mārga*) can be compared to a gigantic organism the individual members of which are exactly fixed in their functioning and sequence of stages, with the teacher (*guru*) as invaluable guidepost. The 'method' of mysticity is commonly 'open' and spontaneous, and the mystic is pre-eminently left to his own resources and is greatly at the mercy of his God whose guiding voice, however, cannot always be clearly heard. The manifest systematic representation of the Yogic path and the invaluable psychological material gathered by the yogins over many centuries accordingly lead to a more conscious, sharper and fuller comprehension of the subtle (*sūkṣma, subtīlis*) aspects of conditioned existence and thus provide better means of securing the realisation of the Unconditioned, the Absolute.

These, then, are the conditions which confront us in traditional Yoga and mysticity. In this form, however, they cannot exhaust the spiritual teaching and practice of Meister Eckehart, the most able religious thinker and seer of the Middle Ages; he leaves both far behind. To appropriately consider and evaluate those metaphysical summits to which Eckehart gained access, we must draw on the loftiest creations of the Indian genius.

Meister Eckehart's philosophy can be understood only from the standpoint of a Yoga that transcends all magic and mysticism and is intellectually well consolidated. Such an advanced form of Yoga is to be found, for example, among the masters of Mahāyāna and Vajrayāna Buddhism. We also happen on it in the new integral or *pūrṇa-yoga* of Śrī Aurobindo, possibly in a more adequate form. The noteworthy feature of this Yoga is its radical lifting up of the opposition between the two basic modalities of existence—transcendence and immanence, unconditioned and conditioned, *nirvāṇa* and *saṃsāra*. In the practical-cum-ethical domain this, in the words of H. Chaudury, has the following consequences:

[6] There exist, however, popular 'Yoga' movements which, like the *bhakti-yoga*, predominantly operate in the emotional sphere and which are in no way superior to any other form of traditional mysticity.

> Having reached the pinnacle of the supramental realisation, the integral yogi is again to descend; he is to come to the point of his departure, to the physical consciousness, and he is to bring down there the light and power of the supramental Truth-Consciousness.[7]

As opposed to this, the Pātañjalayoga is a 'one-way street'. There is an ascent, but no descent. The yogin rests content with realising the Self apart from the phenomenal world. The same view is taken by Śaṅkara who appears to have been unable to reconcile the unmanifested and the manifested aspects of *brahman*.

Meister Eckehart was born about the year 1260, a crucial period in the making of Germany: enormous natural catastrophes accentuated the social need, the 'black death' made its cruel procession, the Church experienced one of its severest crises, heretic movements sprang up eagerly turning against the rigid and sacrilegiously arrogant scholasticism, and fanatic holy wars were fought in the name of God. The people, suffering injustice, suppression and fear, stood face to face with the impermanence of human existence and yearned for a deep spiritual experience which would finally bring them security and foothold. In India it is a common belief that whenever there are times of such darkness and spiritual stagnation, 'great souls' (*mahā-ātmas*) are incarnated to diffuse their light upon all those who, in spite of gloomy surroundings, remain pure in heart and intent. In the *Bhagavad-Gītā*, the famous dialogue between the divine Kṛṣṇa and the royal warrior and spiritual hero Arjuna, the following verse is contained:

> Whenever there is a diminution of the spiritual order (*dharma*), o Bhārata [=Arjuna], and a rise of *adharma*—then I create forth Myself [in form of a *homo nobilis*].[8]

We believe that Eckehart was one such great soul. Like a bright meteor he ascended into the black sky of the Middle Ages, lighting up the horizon with the radiance of his immense transcendental insight and compassion, *prajñā* and *karuṇā*. His message is, as also that of the Indian sages, simple and unequivocal and yet extremely difficult to

[7] H. Chaudury, Śrī *Aurobindo: The Prophet of Life Divine* (Calcutta, 1951), p. 46.

[8] BhG IV.7. *Cf. Bhāgavata-Purāṇa* IX.24.56: 'Whenever there is a [spiritual] decline and an increase of sin here [on earth], the divine lord, Hari, creates himself forth (*sṛjate*).'

comprehend. Eckehart himself was fully aware of this, for at the conclusion of one of his sermons he says:

> He who does not understand this discourse is not to afflict his heart with it. For so long as a man does not resemble this truth, that long he will not understand this discourse. For it is an unveiled truth which has come straight out of the heart of God.[9]

In this passage Eckehart not only repeats the esoteric formula that equal is only recognised by equal, but in it he also expounds his most fundamental axiom: the 'birth of Christ' in the soul, which empowers him to pronounce with unshakable certainty that what he utters is truth, for it was begot in 'the heart of God'. God's word sounds eternally,[10] but it is only in the highest part of the soul that his almighty word is echoed. Consequently, to utter truth means to have lifted oneself up to this summit of existence. That is exactly what Eckehart wants to commit to us. For him, as also for the *vedāntin*, God and man are *essentially* identical. 'God and I, we are one',[11] says the Meister very much in the style of the Upaniṣads. Naturally, he provoked the anger and ill-humour of the clergymen of his time to whom God was something man could never reach. It is thus not at all surprising that this basic tenet of Eckehart's teaching was among the twenty-eight articles condemned as heretical or suspicious of heresy in the bull 'In agro dominico' of Pope John XXII.

The core of one's being, which is identical with the barren Godhead, is beyond any adequate assertion. Like Yājñavalkya, the grand figure of the Upaniṣads, Eckehart makes ample use of negative descriptions. 'God is neither this nor that.'[12] Elsewhere he says: '. . . one must illustrate God by way of similes, with *this* or *that*. Yet he is neither this nor that.'[13] In a well-known passage of the *Bṛhadāraṇyaka-Upaniṣad*, Yājñavalkya declares:

> This Self (*ātman*) is neither this nor that (*neti, neti*). Incomprehensible,

[9] Sermon 6. J. Quint, *Meister Eckehart. Deutsche Predigten und Traktate* (München, 1955).
[10] *Cf. Śatapatha-Brāhmaṇa* II.1.4.10: 'The word is the Absolute' (*vāg vai brahma*).
[11] Sermon 7.
[12] Sermon 10.
[13] Sermon 24.

> it is not to be grasped; indestructible, it is not to be destroyed; non-clinging, it does not cling; not bound, it does not shake.[14]

Yet this realisation did not stop Yājñavalkya from speaking of the Absolute in terms of 'consciousness-bliss' (*cid-ānanda*).[15] Both he and Eckehart were fully aware that in order to impart their knowledge to others, they had to employ a language of either negative, positive or paradoxical terms when referring to the One beyond all definition, the Signless and Nameless. For the benefit of his fellow-beings, Eckehart availed himself of all three possibilities, much to the confusion of some scholars, who discern in his writings only endless contradictions and scholastic quibble.[16] Fortunately, not all Eckehart interpreters show the same lack of insight. Two studies here are of special interest since they were carried out by scholars well acquainteed with Eastern thought; we refer to the respective works by D. T. Suzuki[17] and R. Otto.[18] The former pertinently remarks:

> As far as I can judge, Eckhart[19] seems to be an extraordinary 'Christian'.
>
> While refraining from going into details we can say at least this: Eckhart's Christianity is unique and has many points which make us hesitate to classify him as belonging to the type we generally associate with rationalised modernism or with conservative traditionalism. He stands in his own experiences which emerged from a deep, religious personality.[20]

The present sketch is an attempt to relate some of Eckehart's doctrines to Yoga, that is, to outline the more significant resemblances and differences between them. Two points of agreement have already been cited, namely that (i) man is in essence a transcendent being,

[14] Bṛh. Up. IV.2.4.

[15] *Vide* Bṛh. Up. III.9.28.

[16] Even such a splendid scholar as F. C. Happold repeats in his *Mysticism: A Study and an Anthology*, 2nd impr. (Harmondsworth, 1967), p. 240, the usual unjust criticism that Eckehart 'sometimes indulges in wild exaggeration and paradox'.

[17] D. T. Suzuki, *Mysticism: Christian and Buddhist* (London, 1957).

[18] T. Otto, *Mysticism East and West: A Compatarive analysis of the nature of mysticism*, transl. by B. L. Bracey and R. C. Payne (New York, Collier Books, 1962).

[19] The correct translation of the Latin Ecehardus would be Eckehart.

[20] op. cit., p. 4.

in so far as he is one with the Absolute, and that (ii) therefore the highest aim (*parama-artha*) of human life is to re-establish this original mode of existence, to experience the 'birth of Christ' in the soul. Both axioms are diametrically opposed to the spirit of orthodox Christianity in which God is ever apart from the created cosmos including man. This assumption is, for example, reflected in *The Cloud of Unknowing*:

> . . . there was never yet pure creature in this life, nor never yet shall be, so high ravished in contemplation and love of the Godhead, that there is not evermore a high and a wonderful cloud of unknowing betwixt him and his God.[21]

For the anonymous author, the supreme goal of spiritual life was to come into contact with God and to unite with him (*unio mystica*). But the abyss between creature and creator cannot be bridged and full identification is therefore impossible. Eckehart, his Faustic mind sternly directed towards the Absolute, went beyond such dualism. As Pope John XXII remarked: 'He wanted to know more than is necessary.' Unlike Gregory of Nyssa who taught that man's ascent in itself is the goal, the Meister aspired to the transcendent core itself, the Godhead beyond space and time. Here Eckehart entirely ignores orthodox Christianity, Judaism and Islam in which world and God have their independent existence. He dared to put truth, as he conceived it, before Church dogma. Swimming against the tide, it was inevitable that he should sooner or later be accused of heresy. Yet Eckehart was keen to remain loyal to the Church, as is shown by his defence in matters regarding the accusation of pantheism. Nevertheless he was fully conscious of the danger surrounding him, but he faced it with serenity and possibly even slight amusement, as the following extract from one of his sermons suggests. Leaning on St. Augustine's dictum that 'what a man loves a man is', Eckehart says:

> If he loves a stone he is just that stone, if he loves a man he is that man, if he loves God—nay, I durst not say more; were I to say, he is God, ye might stone me.[22]

[21] Chapter XVII. Ed. by E. Underhill, *A Book of Contemplation the which is called The Cloud of Unknowing in the which a soul is oned with God*, 6th ed. (London, 1956).
[22] F. Pfeiffer, *The Works of Meister Eckehart*, Engl. transl. by C. de B. Evans, 2nd impr. (London, 1947), vol. I, p. 157. (Sermon LXIII.)

The soul is not *like* God, but the very same as he is. He was never tired of preaching about this fundamental one-ness of man and God and of describing that 'noble man' (*homo nobilis*) who has risen to the very height of the spiritual path. 'Such a man is bearing God in all his acts as well as in all places, and all acts of this man God alone does.'[23] Like an ardent lover who, amidst other activities, cares only for his beloved, the 'noble man' carries God alone in his mind in whatever situation. To such a person, God is apparent in all things. Eckehart also characterises this state as a 'standing-in-oneself',[24] the exact Sanskrit equivalent of which is *svarūpa-pratiṣṭhā*, a Yogic term to be found in the *Yoga-Sūtra.*[25] In another of his sermons, he states:

> The man who thus knows all that God knows is a God-knowing man. This man grasps God in his own-being [Sanskrit *sva-bhāva*] and in his own unity and in his own presence as well as in his own truth [Sanskrit *ātma-tattva*].[26]

Evidently, this exalted state is not reached without extreme effort and purification (*κάθαρσις*, *śuddhi*). The person desirous of it must conquer three great obstacles of time, corporeality and multiplicity.[27] In a touching passage Eckehart speaks of the supreme goal in the following words:

> Listen to the wonder! How wonderful: to stand outside as well as in, to grasp and be grasped, to look on and at the same time be the seen itself, to hold and be held—that is the aim.[28]

Having reached the goal, man is no longer conscious of himself. Hence he is also not aware that it is God who works through him and in him. 'How can the knower be known?', asks Yājñavalkya.[29] Although

[23] *Reden der Unterweisung*, §6.
[24] Sermon 3.
[25] *Vide* YS IV.34. This term is a synonym of *kaivalya*, the 'alone-ness' of the liberated yogin.
[26] Sermon 11.
[27] Sermon 12. *Cf. Māṇḍūkya-Up.* I: 'All that which transcends the threefold time (*trikālātīta*) is also the Absolute.' In the text the word 'absolute' is replaced by the sacred syllable *oṃ*.
[28] Sermon 28.
[29] Bṛh. Up. II.4.14.

the Meister held fast to the basic identity of God and soul, he nevertheless let it be understood in a number of his sermons that the soul cannot exhaust God.

> Should a drop be poured into the impetuous ocean, the drop would be turned into the ocean and not the ocean into the drop. Such also is the case with the soul: when God draws it into himself, it is transformed into him, so that the soul is made divine, but not God [made] the soul.[30]

To this there is a striking analogy in the *Bṛhadāraṇyaka-Upaniṣad* where Yājñavalkya instructs his wife, Maitreyī, in the science of non-duality:

> As a lump of salt when thrown into water dissolves into mere water, [and] there would be none to seize it, as it were, because from wherever one might take [water], it would have the taste of salt—thus verily this great being (*mahad-bhūta*) is infinite, boundless, pure knowledge (*vijñāna-ghana*).[31]

Eckehart's conception of the Absolute is very similar to that of the seer-philosopher of the *Śvetāśvatara-Upaniṣad* who affirms:

> In this tremendous wheel of the Absolute (*brahma-cakra*), in which everything lives, in which all stands, the individual [lit. the 'swan' or *haṃsa*] is whirled about, because he conceives the Self as distinct from the inciter. When blessed by Him, he enters immortality (*amṛtatva*).[32]

The Meister's teaching is not merely metaphysics, but metaphysics with soteriological aims, as clearly demonstrated by R. Otto. In other words, it is directed towards the goal of emancipation through a realisation of the 'naked Being' (*nudum esse*), the barren Godhead. This liberation, the *summum bonum* of human life, is but the awareness of one's eternal freedom. For the Self, the *bürgelin*, was never born into the cycle of cosmic becoming and disbecoming, but stood in absolute

[30] Sermon 55.
[31] Bṛh. Up. II.4.12. *Cf. Kaṭha-Up.* IV.14, *Muṇḍaka-Up.* III.2.8 and Śaṅkara's *Viveka-Cūḍāmaṇi* 566.
[32] Śvet. Up. I.6.

purity from all eternity. Thus realisation (*anubhava*) is simply the removal of ignorance (*avidyā*). This is the view of Yoga and Vedānta and is also held by Eckehart. With the realisation of the One-without-a-second (*ekam-advitīyam*) arises true knowledge (*vidyā*)˙ or, more accurately, Self-realisation *is* pure awareness, supreme knowledge.

Eckehart undeniably experienced the most profound enstatic (*samādhi*) states.[33] These, however, were not the result of mere accident or gratification, but the result of protracted and consistent spiritual practice. This is not only illustrated by the sublimity and the psychological penetration of his thought, but also by the fact that he was a Dominican monk to whom contemplation and other spiritual exercises were a part of daily life. And yet R. Otto alleged that it is peculiar to Eckehart's teaching that, quite contrary to Luther, he recognised no *methodus operandi*. Comparing Śaṅkara's and Eckehart's spiritual philosophy, he states:

> Their method is the same, it consists in this—that in reality they have none! All that we usually term 'mystical method', all purposeful self-training for 'mystical experiences,' all soul-direction, schooling, exercising, the technique of attaining a spiritual state, artificial exaltation of the Self—this is far removed from them and lies aside from their path.[34]

This claim, as it stands, does not appear to receive much support from the writings of both masters themselves. Emphasising the importance of the doctrinal or intellectual aspect in both teachings, R. Otto shows less attentiveness and *Tiefblick* with regard to the practical side of the two paths. Spiritual life is a bi-polar affair. Man ascends by swinging alternately between the two poles of 'death' and 'rebirth'. The former, the negative aspect, represents man's effort to obliterate the 'old Adam', the latter, the positive aspect, his endeavour to experience spiritual resurrection. Any system which aims at a spiritual renewal of man has to take this into account. Without these two poles no spiritual ascent (ἀνάβασις) is possible. *Via illuminativa* (*pravṛtti-mārga*) in itself is devoid of the power of spiritual uplift. Just so, *via negativa* (*nivṛtti-mārga*), without the positive remoulding of man, cannot lead to the

[33] *Cf.* D. T. Suzuki, *Mysticism: Christian and Buddhist*, p. 79: '. . . I am sure Eckehart had a *satori*.'
[34] R. Otto, *Mysticism East and West*, p. 47.

final goal. Only when *abhyāsa* (the constructive unification practice) and *vairāgya* (the effort at dismantling human personality) are practised together and assist each other can true progress take place. In the *Bhagavad-Gītā* we find:

> Doubtlessly, o strong-armed [Arjuna], the mind is fickle and hard to be checked. But, o son of Kuntī, it can be seized by *abhyāsa* and *vairāgya*.[35]

Naturally, both aspects of spiritual life require the same amount of attention from the *sādhaka*, yogin or mystic. Unless he realises that *abhyāsa* and *vairāgya* complement each other, he is likely to fall prey to either 'mystical' revelling and hallucinatory visions (when his renunciation is not supported by the purifying effect of concentration) or to the magical powers (*siddhis*) gained by his practice of concentration, but not neutralised by *vairāgya*. In both cases the fruits of his 'spiritual' efforts fall on unprepared ground and produce abnormal ego disintegration in the one instance and pathological egocentricism and arrogance in the other. By nature, the plus-pole, *abhyāsa*, is open to more detailed treatment and elaboration than *vairāgya*. The yogins have made ample use of this fact, and the systematic development of this aspect is perhaps the most striking feature of Yoga.

Although it is correct that Eckehart's writings, like those of Śaṅkara, contain very little instruction as to the *pravṛtti* element of the path, this must not, as R. Otto supposes, necessarily mean that 'the technique for attaining a spiritual state' lies outside their scheme of emancipation. Śaṅkara was always held in highest esteem not only as a philosopher, but also as a yogin. Numerous legends, to this effect, have been woven around his name. His popular works, like the *Viveka-Cūḍāmaṇi* and the *Aparokṣa-Anubhūti*, too, seem to contradict Otto's view.

Eckehart's position, however, is slightly more intricate. First of all, there is insufficient material at our disposal to make a definite claim that Eckehart had no 'mystical method'. Little is known about his career and almost nothing about his more personal life. Otto's assumption rests entirely on a study of the sermons, treatises and other writings. The following observations can here be made. Unlike Śaṅkara, the Meister had a public which was little acquainted with the deeper elements of spiritual life. While Eckehart intended his Latin

[35] BhG VI.35.

works for the learned of his day who expressed a keen interest in metaphysical speculation, while remaining decidedly aloof with regard to spiritual practice, the German writings were directed especially at the lay masses. In both instances, Eckehart had no illusions about the amount of understanding he would receive. He thought it pointless even to begin to indicate the details of the techniques of unification. This could only have led to even greater confusion and stronger adverse criticism. He confined himself to an outline of his basic philosophy and stressed renunciation (*gelāzenheit*), the negative pole of the path, the principles of which can be understood and practised by anyone. He only imparted the positive aspect to those pupils who had sufficient motivation (*mumukṣutva*, the desire for liberation) and power of concentration to attempt the practice of unification. However, some traces of Eckehart's practical experience and teaching are to be found in his works:

> The divine light cannot shine into them [*i.e.* into the forces of the soul]; yet through exercise and chastening they can become receptive.[36]

> . . . collect your senses, all your powers, your entire reason and all your memory: direct these into that core wherein this treasure lies hidden.[37]

Both quotations, in our opinion, clearly contravene Otto's strange assumption. The second excerpt is of special interest, since it contains a statement of the consecutive stages of the withdrawal of the senses (*pratyāhāra*), concentration (*dhāraṇā*) and meditation (*dhyāna*). It is most probable that the mention of the phrase 'memory' refers to the latter.

As Otto has shown in the light of numerous quotations from Eckehart's work, the Meister experienced the extrovertive type of enstasis (*saṃprajñāta-samādhi*) as well as the introvertive (*asaṃprajñāta-*). He had attained to the *visio mundi* as well as the *visio dei*. In the first the cosmos is beheld in one act as a whole (*sarvatā*) wherein all opposites coincide, perfect identity in difference. This experience of unity grows progressively stronger, till the One has become a '*real* above the many',

[36] Sermon 11.
[37] Sermon 58.

as Otto characterises the third stage of this process of unification.[38] The second type of enstasis is devoid of any object; it is a purely subjective state in which the Self, the pure subject, illumines itself in itself and by itself. As the Meister puts it: 'Then God is recognised by God in the soul.'[39]

Apparently having had no instructor, this outstanding attainment bears full witness to Eckehart's genius. Like Rāmana, the great seer-yogin of Tiruvannamalai, he had found truth solely by relying on the 'inner guide' (*antaryāmin*), the *guru* within his own heart. Unknowingly, the Dominican monk of the 13-14th century has followed the advice given by Gautama, the founder of Buddhism, some eighteen hundred years earlier, when he bade his disciples to be 'lamps unto themselves, refuge to themselves'.[40]

So far it was our endeavour to accentuate the resemblances between Eckehart's teaching and that of the two great representatives of Vedānta on the one hand and Yoga on the other. But, as Otto has boldly set forth, there is one prominent point of difference between the *darśanas* of Śaṅkara and Patañjali and Eckehart's doctrine: For the two Eastern masters, liberation consists in a total withdrawal from the sphere of human activities and, indeed, from the world (*saṃsāra*) as such, whilst Eckehart—to whom the Absolute is not static, but infinitely dynamic, the 'living God'—preaches of a divine life here and now, since 'God is in all creatures equally close'.[41]

However, Otto's attempt to draw a sharp distinction between the two eminent masters (*ācārya*=Meister) of Oriental and Occidental mysticity with regard to their respective conceptions of emancipation and God is to be looked upon with some reservation. It is true that Eckehart's statements about the Absolute convey pre-eminently the impression of a dynamic, living 'process', while the works of Śaṅkara manifestedly emphasise the idea of a static, immovable, serene 'being'.[42] Yet Otto's tendency to regard the transcendental realisations of the two seer-philosophers as *factually* differing is not without its dangers.

[38] R. Otto, *Mysticism East and West*, p. 70.
[39] Sermon 1.
[40] *Mahā-Parinibbāṇa-Sutta* II.33.
[41] Sermon 36.
[42] Already the equalisation of *brahman* with *ānanda* suggests a certain degree of vitalism in Śaṅkara's conception of the Absolute.

We must bear in mind that the ideas of dynamism and static are *interpretations* only, determined by the prevailing disposition of the individual, attributions to the One beyond the grasp of the mind, not actual experiences. Furthermore, to the perfected being (*siddha*) two ways are open: either the way of active life or that of withdrawal. The possibility of the one does not exclude the other. There is at least one passage in Śaṅkara's *Bhāṣya* to the *Brahma-Sūtra* of Bādarāyaṇa, the classical manual of Vedānta, which evinces that the *ācārya* was quite conscious of the fact that there were these two possibilities, though he naturally tended to give prominence to his own point of view.[43] In his commentary to *sūtra* IV.3.14 of Bādarāyaṇa's textbook he announces that

> practical life will hold its place even then [when the Self is realised], just as dreamlife holds its place up to the moment of waking.[44]

Both Śaṅkara and Eckehart agree on the principal issue of the problem of how it is possible that the liberated person can live in the world and perform actions without becoming re-involved in the cycle of phenomenal existence. The former teacher declares in his *Viveka-Cūḍāmaṇi*, a very readable popular exposition of Advaita-Vedānta:

> He who never has the thought of 'I' with regard to the body and the senses and the thought of 'this' in respect of something different to the *tat* [the Absolute], is regarded as a *jīvan-mukta*.[45]

Such a man is, as the *Chāndogya-Upaniṣad* affirms, like a lotus flower not defiled by the muddy water surrounding it.[46] Eckehart visualises an *active* life founded on the realisation of the Self. The basic principle of his teaching is: to give out in love what has been gathered in contemplation. His aim was not to undergo ecstatic or even enstatic experiences, but to realise unitive life, of which E. Underhill says:

[43] *Vide Brahma-Sūtra-Bhāṣya* III.4.13, 14. *Cf.* also III.3.32 where he discusses those cases of liberated beings who, like Apāntaratamas, Vaśiṣṭha, Bhṛgu, Sanatkumāra, Dakṣa, and Nārada took on a new body to fulfill a mission (*adhikāra*).

[44] In other passages of his great commentary, Śaṅkara takes a more radical view.

[45] Verse 438. *Cf.* Śaṅkara's *Ātmabodha* 46, 49 and 50. Also *Viveka Cūḍāmaṇi*, 431–7 and 439.

[46] *Vide* Chānd. Up. IV.14.3.

> . . . though so often lived in the world, is never of it. It belongs to another plane of being, moves securely upon levels unrelated to our speech; and hence eludes the measuring powers of humanity. We, from the valley, can only catch a glimpse of the true life of these elect spirits, transfigured upon the mountain. They are far away, breathing another air: we cannot reach them. Yet it is impossible to over-estimate their importance for the race. They are our ambassadors of the Absolute.[47]

Eckehart formulates his exact standpoint thus:

> That a man has a peaceful or reposing life in God—that is good; that a man bears a troublesome life with patience—that is better; but that one has peace in a troublesome life—that is the best of all.[48]

Accordingly, the sign of the God-realised man is not the number of days he is able to spend in *samādhi* or the size of his following, but the attitude he shows towards his fellow-beings. Eckehart's ethics demand that such a person should quite willingly interrupt his contemplation, however deep and exalted it may be, if an ill or a poor person was in need.[49] The Meister's logic behind this is simple:

> If you love bliss more in yourself than in another, you [only] love yourself; and where you love yourself, there God is not your pure love, and that is wrong.[50]

For Eckehart, it was the active Martha and not the contemplative Maria, sitting at the feet of the master Jesus, who had reached a higher degree of perfection.[51] The perfected being stands outside and inside all things, he is perceiver and perceived at once. He does not cease performing acts and duties, but accepts life as a manifestation of the divine. Having reached the Self, the soul's core, which is realised as One and thus as non-different from the cosmos, the transformed being turns back to the world, now acting as a connecting link between the

[47] E. Underhill, *Mysticism: A Study in the Nature and Development of Man's Spiritual Consciousness,* 1st ed. 1911, repr. (London, 1957), p. 414.

[48] Sermon 36.

[49] *Reden der Unterweisung* §10.

[50] Sermon 43.

[51] Sermon 28.

transcendent and the empirical universe, thus in himself reconciling both aspects of reality.

This is in full harmony with the doctrines of Mahāyāna Buddhism according to which *saṃsāra* (the phenomenal world) and *nirvāṇa* are but two designations of one and the same reality. As resolutely stated in Nāgārjuna's *Mādhyamika-Śāstra*:

> There is no difference at all
> between *nirvāṇa* and *saṃsāra*.
> There is no difference at all
> between *saṃsāra* and *nirvāṇa*.[52]

This realisation is not a mere intellectual operation, but a transcendental act which induces a total change within the individual enabling him to 'live' in both orders of existence, transcendental and phenomenal. However, this does not mean that he perceives the empirical cosmos and the transcendent at the same time. There can only be experience of the one or the other. In Haṭhayoga this fact finds expression in the statement that when the 'serpent power', *kuṇḍalinī*, 'sleeps' in man, he is awake, but when it is awake, he loses awareness of the phenomenal world, abiding in pure consciousness and supreme bliss. The puzzling state of duality in non-duality in the perfected being (*siddha*) presupposes an absolute elasticity of the psychomental framework of the person in question in order to receive the 'impulses' of the transcendent Self undistortedly and yet being fully aware of the empirical environment.

The ethics advocated by Eckehart are foreshadowed by the *Īśa-Upaniṣad* and taught in full by the *Bhagavad-Gītā*. In the latter scripture the God-teacher Kṛṣṇa propounds to his disciple Arjuna one of the profoundest doctrines brought forth on Indian soil:

> No one ever remains, even for an instant (*kṣaṇa*), without performing action (*karma*). Everyone is will-lessly forced to act, by the primary energies (*guṇas*) of nature.
>
> A person does not obtain actionlessness (*naiṣkarmya*) by abstention from work, and he does also not come to perfection (*siddhi*) by mere renunciation (*saṃnyāsa*).[53]

[52] XXV.19. The translation is that of Stcherbatsky.
[53] BhG III.5 and III.4.

And the divine *guru*, giving himself as an example, proceeds:

> For me, o Pārtha [*i.e.* Arjuna], there is nothing to be done in the three worlds, nothing to be obtained which has not [already] been obtained—and yet I continue with [performing] work.[54]
>
> If I should fail to perform action, these worlds (*lokas*) would perish, and I would be the author of chaos (*saṃkara*) and destroy these creatures.[55]

This is exactly the Christian conception of the 'living God', beautifully reflected in Eckehart's statement that 'God tastes himself in all things'.[56] Having proclaimed the universal validity of action, Kṛṣṇa continues:

> . . . Though I am the author (*kartṛ*) of it [*i.e.* of the fourfold social order etc.], know Me to be the non-author, immutable.
>
> Action does not stain Me, nor do I have longing (*spṛhā*) for action's fruit. He who experiences Me thus is not bound by work.[57]

Then the godly teacher reveals the secret of inaction in action (*akarma-karma*):

> He who in action sees inaction and inaction in action is enlightened among men, is a *yukta* [or yogin of the highest order] performing all work (*kṛtsna-karma-kṛt*).
>
> [He whose] works are consumed in the fire of [true] knowledge (*jñāna*), him the sages call a knower (*paṇḍita*).
>
> Having renounced his clinging to the fruit of action, forever satisfied, without [foreign] support, he, though occupied with work, does not do anything at all.[58]

[54] BhG III.22.
[55] BhG III.24.
[56] Sermon 26.
[57] BhG IV.13 and 14.
[58] BhG IV.18–20.

> [He who] has renounced [all] action by Yoga, has cut asunder doubt (*saṃśaya*) by knowledge and is self-controlled [or possessed by the Self]—him no action can bind, o conqueror of spiritual wealth![59]

Arjuna then enquires from the lord:

> O Kṛṣṇa, you praise renunciation (*saṃnyāsa*) of [all] action and then again Yoga. Which one of these two is more excellent? That tell me for certain![60]

The divine teacher replies:

> Renunciation [of all action] and the Yoga of action are both inducive of the *summum bonum* (*niḥśreyas*). But of these two [paths], *karmayoga* is superior to [mere] renunciation of [all] action.[61]

The ideal of *naiṣkarmya* or actionlessness in action strictly opposes any attempt at a *Weltflucht*, a fleeing from the responsibilities of life. Yet, as is evident from Kṛṣṇa's discourse, complete renunciation of all work is not wrong, but also leads to the final absorption in the Absolute. However, he leaves no doubt about the fact that full acceptance of life, combined with a detachment from one's activities and a complete renunciation of their fruits on the basis of perfect Self-realisation, is infinitely superior to a simple withdrawal from the world. This is entirely in agreement with Eckehart's views. Speaking of the attainment of transcendental love (*karuṇā*), he declares:

> He who is caught in this snare [of divine love] and who walks this path, whatever work he performs or does not perform, is of one kind; it is completely irrelevant whether he is doing something or not. And yet, such a man's most trifling work or exercise is, for himself and mankind, more useful and fruitful and more pleasing to God than the exercises of all those men who, though free from mortal sins, have lesser love. His leisure is more profitable than another's work.[62]

[59] BhG IV.41.
[60] BhG V.1.
[61] BhG V.2.
[62] Sermon 59.

Elsewhere the Meister states:

> The wiser and mightier a master is, the more spontaneously is carried out his work and the simpler it is.[63]

The man who succeeded in reaching 'the uppermost top' (*daz oberste wipfellîn*) of his soul, the Self, can pronounce with utter certainty: 'My work is not *my* work, my life is not *my* life.'[64] For he has ceased to have a human personality, with all the limitations peculiar to it, but thinks and acts spontaneously from the centre of his being, his thought or non-thought, doing or non-doing being determined only by the transcendental powers of *prajñā* and *karuṇā.*

> The righteous man (*gerehte mensch*) serves neither God nor creatures, *for he is free.*[65]

[63] Sermon 57.
[64] Sermon 38.
[65] Sermon 31.

Diagram I: The ontological elements of Pātañjalayoga

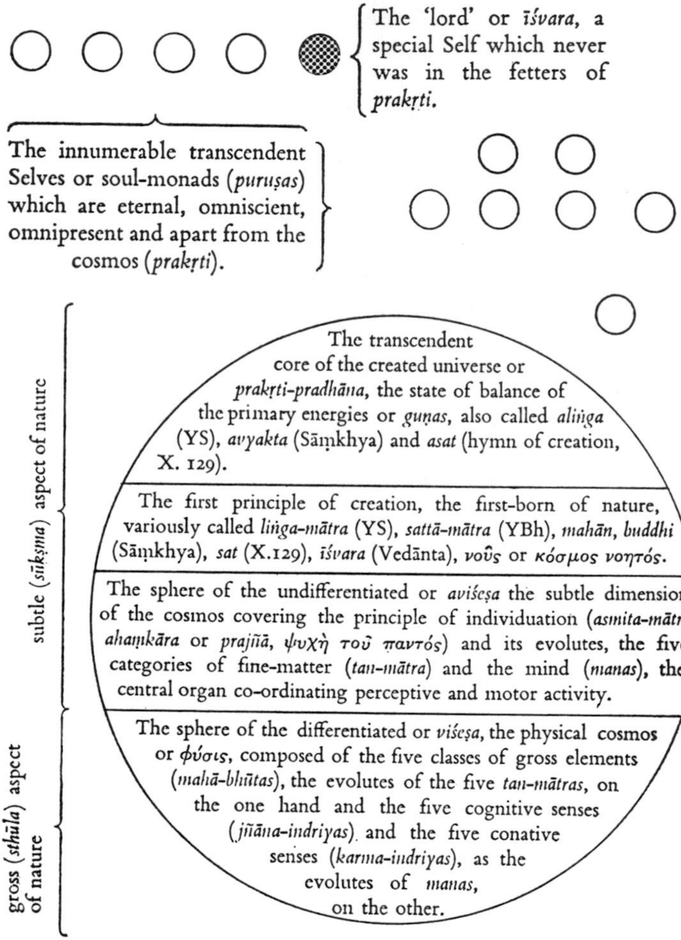

The 'lord' or *īśvara*, a special Self which never was in the fetters of *prakṛti*.
The innumerable transcendent Selves or soul-monads (*puruṣas*) which are eternal, omniscient, omnipresent and apart from the cosmos (*prakṛti*).
subtle (*sūkṣma*) aspect of nature
gross (*sthūla*) aspect of nature
The transcendent core of the created universe or *prakṛti-pradhāna*, the state of balance of the primary energies or *guṇas*, also called *aliṅga* (YS), *avyakta* (Sāṃkhya) and *asat* (hymn of creation, X. 129).
The first principle of creation, the first-born of nature, variously called *liṅga-mātra* (YS), *sattā-mātra* (YBh), *mahān*, *buddhi* (Sāṃkhya), *sat* (X.129), *īśvara* (Vedānta), *νοῦς* or *κόσμος νοητός*.
The sphere of the undifferentiated or *aviśeṣa* the subtle dimension of the cosmos covering the principle of individuation (*asmita-mātra*, *ahaṃkāra* or *prajñā*, *ψυχὴ τοῦ παντός*) and its evolutes, the five categories of fine-matter (*tan-mātra*) and the mind (*manas*), the central organ co-ordinating perceptive and motor activity.
The sphere of the differentiated or *viśeṣa*, the physical cosmos or *φύσις*, composed of the five classes of gross elements (*mahā-bhūtas*), the evolutes of the five *tan-mātras*, on the one hand and the five cognitive senses (*jñāna-indriyas*) and the five conative senses (*karma-indriyas*), as the evolutes of *manas*, on the other.

Diagram II: The stages of enstasis (*samādhi*) according to the *Yoga-Sūtra* of Patañjali

emancipation
or
kaivalya

▲

dharma-megha-samādhi

the enstasis bringing about the involution of the primary energies (*guṇas*) of nature and thus leading to immediate liberation; the causes of bondage and suffering, *i.e.* the fruits of *karma* and the *kleśas* in form of subconscious residua (*saṃskāras*) are exterminated; all is mastered (*sarva-nirodha*)

▲

asaṃprajñāta-samādhi

the enstasis procured by supreme abandonment (*para-vairāgya*) of all wordly objects; it is devoid of any awarenesses (*pratyayas*); only subconscious impressions (*saṃskāras*) are left which, through repeated practice, are burnt up

▲

viveka-khyāti

the uninterrupted discriminative vision between the Self and the world, also referred to as *puruṣa-khyāti*, *vivekaja-jñāna* and *tāraka-jñāna*;

▲

asmitā-samādhi

the enstasis connected with the awareness of oneself, probably a phase of *nirvicāra-samādhi*

▲

ānanda-samādhi

the enstasis connected with supreme joy, probably a subdivision of *nirvicāra samādhi*

▲

nirvicāra-samādhi

the enstasis having a subtle (*sūkṣma*) object as support and being devoid of any supramental 'reflection' or *vicāra*

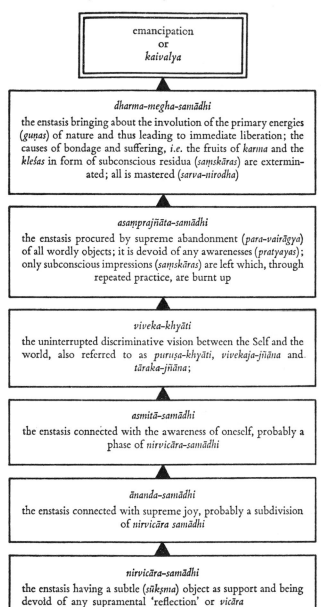

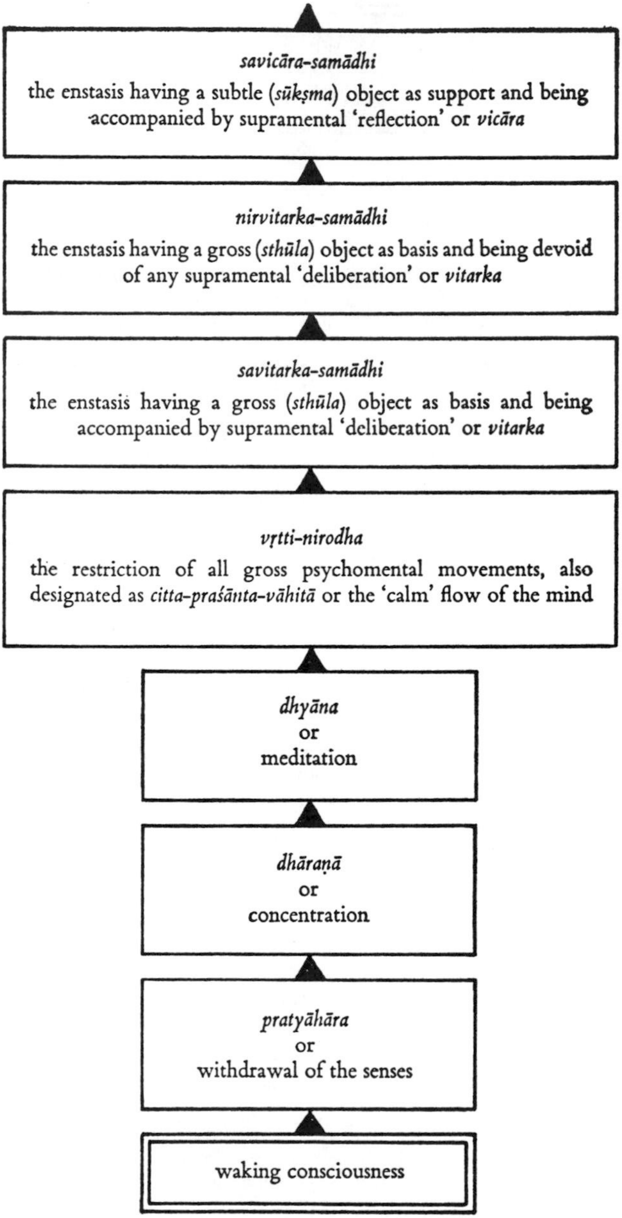
savicāra-samādhi
the enstasis having a subtle (*sūkṣma*) object as support and being accompanied by supramental 'reflection' or *vicāra*
nirvitarka-samādhi
the enstasis having a gross (*sthūla*) object as basis and being devoid of any supramental 'deliberation' or *vitarka*
savitarka-samādhi
the enstasis having a gross (*sthūla*) object as basis and being accompanied by supramental 'deliberation' or *vitarka*
vṛtti-nirodha
the restriction of all gross psychomental movements, also designated as *citta-praśānta-vāhitā* or the 'calm' flow of the mind
dhyāna
or
meditation
dhāraṇā
or
concentration
pratyāhāra
or
withdrawal of the senses
waking consciousness

Index